Ethical Decision Making in
NURSING
ADMINISTRATION

Mary Cipriano Silva, PhD, RN, FAAN
Professor
School of Nursing
George Mason University
Fairfax, Virginia

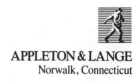

APPLETON & LANGE
Norwalk, Connecticut

0-8385-2469-9

Copyright © 1990 by Appleton & Lange
A Publishing Division of Prentice Hall

90 91 92 93 94 / 10 9 8 7 6 5 4 3 2 1

Prentice Hall International (UK) Limited, *London*
Prentice Hall of Australia Pty. Limited, *Sydney*
Prentice Hall Canada, Inc., *Toronto*
Prentice Hall Hispanoamericana, S.A., *Mexico*
Prentice Hall of India Private Limited, *New Delhi*
Prentice Hall of Japan, Inc., *Tokyo*
Simon & Schuster Asia Pte. Ltd., *Singapore*
Editora Prentice Hall do Brasil Ltda., *Rio de Janeiro*
Prentice Hall, *Englewood Cliffs, New Jersey*

Library of Congress Cataloging-in-Publication Data

Ethical decision making in nursing administration / [edited by] Mary
  Cipriano Silva.
    p. cm.
  ISBN 0-8385-2469-9
    1. Nursing services—Administration—Decision making. 2. Nursing
ethics. I. Silva, Mary Cipriano.
    [DNLM: 1. Decision Making. 2. Ethics, Nursing. 3. Nursing—
organization and administration. WY 105 E84]
  RT89.E77 1990
  174'.2—dc20
  DNLM/DLC   89-6681
  for Library of Congress   CIP

Acquisitions Editors: Janet Foltin & Stu Horton
Production Editor: Amanda D. Egan
Cover Designer: Janice Barsevich

PRINTED IN THE UNITED STATES OF AMERICA

To my family and friends
For being there

Contents

Contributors

ABOUT THE AUTHOR

Mary Cipriano Silva received her BSN and MS from the Ohio State University and her PhD from the University of Maryland. In 1981 she was a recipient of a National Endowment for the Humanities Award to study ethics at the Kennedy Institute of Ethics, Georgetown University. During 1983–1984 she was a recipient of a Kennedy Fellowship in Medical Ethics for Nursing Faculty, and during May of 1987 she was a Visiting Scholar at The Hastings Center. In addition, she has attended both the basic and advanced bioethics courses at the Kennedy Institute of Ethics. From February 1984 through June 1989, Dr Silva served as Project Director on a Special Project Grant funded by the Division of Nursing, Department of Health and Human Services; this grant focused on "Continuing Education in Ethical Decision Making for Nurse Executives." Dr Silva is a Professor in the School of Nursing at George Mason University, Fairfax, Virginia.

ABOUT THE CHAPTER CONTRIBUTORS

Doris Mueller Goldstein received her BA and MA from the University of Nebraska and her MLS from the University of Maryland. Prior to her appointment in 1973 as the first librarian of the Ethics Library of the Kennedy Institute of Ethics, Georgetown University, Ms Goldstein served in Ethiopia as a Peace Corps Volunteer and worked at the Library of Congress. In 1981 she was appointed Director of Library and Information Services at the Kennedy Institute. In that capacity she coordinates the Institute's information activities, including the National Reference Center for Bioethics Literature and the Bioethics Information Retrieval Project, both supported by the National Library of Medicine. Her publications include an annotated bibliography entitled *Bioethics: A Guide to Information Sources,* published by Gale Research Company in 1982.

Doreen Connor Harper is an Associate Professor of Nursing at George Mason University in Fairfax, Virginia where she coordinates the Adult/Gerontological Nurse Practitioner graduate program. She was formerly Department Chairperson at the University of Maryland School of Nursing, Baltimore County Campus. Dr Harper holds a master's degree in psychiatric nursing, and a PhD in gerontology and primary care of adults. She has developed an interest in ethics as it relates to justice and the delivery of care through her fifteen years of administrative, clinical, and teaching experience.

Helen M. Jenkins received her BSN from the University of Virginia, her MSN from the Catholic University of America, and her PhD from the University of Maryland. She has attended both the basic and the advanced bioethics courses at the Kennedy Institute of Ethics. In addition, during May of 1987 she was a Visiting Scholar at The Hastings Center. Dr Jenkins has written about ethical issues and has presented several papers on ethics in community health nursing. She is an Associate Professor in the School of Nursing, George Mason University.

Mary Graney Trainor received her BSN, MSN and PhD from the Catholic University of America. In 1983 she attended the Intensive Bioethics Course at the Kennedy Institute of Ethics. She is an Associate Professor in the School of Nursing, George Mason University, and teaches bioethics there.

ABOUT THE CHAPTER CASE CONTRIBUTORS AND COMMENTATORS

Clara Adams-Ender received a baccalaureate degree in nursing, a master's degree in medical–surgical nursing, and a master's degree in military art and science. A 27-year veteran of the Army, Brigadier General Adams-Ender is the current Chief of the Army Nurse Corps, Washington, D.C. She has held diverse positions as Chief Nurse, Department of Nursing, Walter Reed Army Medical Center; Inspector General; Assistant Professor of Nursing, University of Maryland; and Chief, Army Nurse Recruitment. She has received numerous medals and commendations from the military and national organizations.

Janet L. Chapin serves as Administrator for Underserved Women in the American College of Obstetricians and Gynecologists in Washington, D.C. Ms Chapin has an associate degree in nursing, a bachelor's degree in philosophy, and a master's degree in public health. Ms Chapin has served in several administrative positions in public health agencies and health care associations.

Ruby E. Elmore, RN, MSN, received her BSN from the University of Maryland and her MSN from the Catholic University of America. Her professional career spanned 34 years at Saint Elizabeth's Hospital, Washington, D.C., where she started out as a staff nurse and eventually rose to Division Chief Nurse. Although she retired as of September 1987, she is active in many professional organizations, including the American Nurses' Association, Black Nurses' Association, and the Mental Health Association of the District of Columbia.

Beth R. Kleb, RN, graduated from Temple University School of Nursing and is currently an administrator at the Fairfax Nursing Center, Fairfax, Virginia. She is a Licensed Nursing Home Administrator, and a member of the American College of Nursing Home Administrators and the Society of Law and Medicine.

Jacqueline Muir, RN, MSN, is Assistant Vice President for Nursing and Operations at Children's Hospital National Medical Center, Washington, D.C. She is also pursuing doctoral studies at George Mason University, Fairfax, Virginia. Ms Muir has a long-held interest in ethical issues related to health care and has formed a multidisciplinary ethics study group. She is a member of Children's Hospital's Institutional Ethics Committee.

Ruby Van Croft, RN, MS, is Director for Special Programs, Visiting Nurse Association, Washington, D.C. In addition to her present position, she has held several other positions at the Visiting Nurse Association, including those of staff nurse, supervisor, and Assistant Director for Contracts and Grants. She received her diploma from Freedman's School of Nursing, her BS from Columbia Union College, and her MS from the University of Maryland.

ABOUT THE APPENDIX CASE CONTRIBUTORS

JoAnne M. Jorgenson, RN, MPH, is Director of Nursing Services, Fairfax County Health Department, Fairfax, Virginia.

Sheila M. McCarthy, RN, MSN, CNAA, is Director of Nursing, The George Washington University Medical Center, Washington, D.C.

Gail Dempsey Russell, RN, MSN, is Vice President/Nursing, Potomac Hospital, Woodbridge, Virginia.

Karen Walborn, RN, MN, is presently Nurse Manager, Hebrew Home of Greater Washington, Rockville, Maryland.

Helen Wilmarth, RN, MSN, is Director Nursing Services at Holy Cross Hospital, Silver Spring, Maryland.

Acknowledgments

The only gift is a portion of thyself.
Ralph Waldo Emerson

I am grateful to many who contributed to this book. First and foremost, I thank the Division of Nursing, Department of Health and Human Services, for the five years of funding that made the Special Project Grant on "Continuing Education in Ethical Decision Making for Nurse Executives" a reality. In particular, deep appreciation goes to Ayeliffe Lenihan, Special Project Grant consultant, who gave this project and book her unfailing support. In addition, special thanks go to Rita Carty, Dean, School of Nursing, George Mason University and to the Graduate School, George Mason University: Each provided me with the time to write—the former through a flexible work schedule and the latter through a Faculty Study Leave.

Others also contributed immensely to this book through critical analysis and chapter and case contributions. Tom L. Beauchamp of The Kennedy Institute reviewed the first six chapters of the book twice, making valuable, thought-provoking, and constructive comments. In addition, Daniel Rothbart of George Mason's Department of Philosophy carefully reviewed Chapter 7, and Gladys White of the Office of Technology Assessment, United States Congress, carefully reviewed Chapter 8. These latter two chapters are written, respectively, by Mary Trainor and Doreen Harper. I owe them, as well as Helen Jenkins, who coauthored Chapter 6 with me, and Doris Goldstein, who authored Appendix A, a debt of gratitude for their contributions to this book and for their loyal colleagueship. Special thanks also go to the nurse administrators who are case contributors and/or case commentators; this book could not have been written without their willingness to share experiences that were often difficult and painful. These nurse administrators are: Clara Adams-Ender, Janet Chapin, Ruby Elmore, JoAnne Jorgenson, Beth Kleb, Sheila McCarthy, Jacqueline Muir, Gail Russell, Ruby Van Croft, Karen Walborn, and Helen Wilmarth.

Support also came from editors, staff, family, and friends. Stu

Horton, former Editor of Nursing, Appleton & Lange, encouraged me to write the book and guided me in its early development, whereas Janet Walsh Foltin, Nursing Editor, and Amanda Egan, Production Editor, saw the book to its completion. Word processing of the book, as well as its many revisions, was done by many excellent and dedicated staff, including Donna Hancock, Maribel Gozé, Graciela Jones, Mary Krauss, and the Office Support Services Department at George Mason University. Finally, my deepest gratitude goes to my family and friends for their loyal support and steadfast interest in this book. To all those previously recognized, as well as to all others who contributed to this book, I offer thanks and thanks again.

Preface

Over the past two decades, advances in science and technology have precipitated serious ethical dilemmas in health care. Although the nursing profession has risen to the challenge of addressing many of these dilemmas, it has remained largely silent in addressing ethical dilemmas in the area of nursing administration. In recently compiled computer searches using MEDLINE and BIOETHICSLINE, I was able to locate only a handful of references that specifically focused on ethics in nursing administration.

This result is troubling in light of the frequency with which nurse administrators deal with ethical issues. During 1986 I asked the 96 members of the Virginia Organization of Nurse Executives to participate in a survey on ethical dilemmas in nursing administration. Of the 65 members who responded to the survey, 58 said that they had recently been involved in resolving one or more ethical dilemmas related to nursing administration; yet few felt highly knowledgeable or self-confident in dealing with these dilemmas. Although the number of participants in the study was small, there is little reason to believe that the data would look different with other groups of nurse administrators.

Thus this book was written to increase nurse administrators' knowledge about and self-confidence in resolving ethical dilemmas. Specifically, the book's purposes are: (1) to provide nurse administrators with basic theoretical knowledge about ethics, and (2) to analyze ethical dilemmas in nursing administration through use of a systematic framework. The book's primary audiences are practicing nurse administrators in all settings and graduate students enrolled in master's or doctoral programs in nursing administration. Because many ethical dilemmas in nursing administration have a clinical component, the book is also appropriate for staff nurses.

In a series of ethics conferences funded by the Division of Nursing from February 1984 through June 1989, I asked nurse administrators to write about ethical dilemmas they had experienced as administrators.

Examples from these writings comprise the case material in this book. I believe these cases are representative of the type and complexity of ethical dilemmas faced by today's nurse administrators.

To analyze ethical dilemmas such as the preceding, nurse administrators need knowledge. How much knowledge is no simple matter, however, and each chapter of this book has gone through many revisions in an effort to strike a balance between content that is neither too simple nor too complex. For those readers who prefer more extensive or varied content, I recommend the references and resources described in Appendix A.

With the preceding overview in mind, the book is organized as follows: Chapters 1 through 4 are theory oriented and Chapters 5 through 8 are application oriented. The theory oriented chapters focus on ethical theories, principles, and moral development. The application oriented chapters focus on application of the preceding content to ethical dilemmas faced by today's nurse administrators.

In addressing the needs of nurse administrators, this book has a number of unique features. First, all ethics cases presented in the book are written by nurse administrators who have dealt with them in their administrative practices. Second, each case analysis is commented on by the nurse administrator who wrote the case. Third, the presented cases are assessed in considerably more depth than those found in most ethics books. Fourth, important points of the book have been highlighted. In sum, every effort has been made to produce a book that is useful for the busy nurse administrator who is attempting to analyze and resolve ethical dilemmas in nursing administration with knowledge, self-confidence, and integrity.

Mary Cipriano Silva
Fairfax, VA

PART I

Theory

Part I of this book contains basic theoretical content needed to analyze ethical dilemmas in nursing administration. To that end, Chapter 1 focuses on two important terms: ethics and ethical dilemmas. Chapter 2 focuses on the classical ethical theories of utilitarianism and deontology. Chapter 3 focuses on the ethical principles of autonomy, beneficence, and justice. Chapter 4 focuses on decision making, values, and stages of moral development as these relate to nursing.

The goal in Part I is to present the preceding theory in a manner that is neither too simple nor too complex. By finding this middle ground, nurse administrators should be able to realistically apply the preceding theory to their administrative practices.

Ethics and Ethical Dilemmas

Mary Cipriano Silva

The simplest questions are the
hardest to answer.
Northrop Frye

In this chapter, two terms essential for understanding ethical decision making are defined: ethics and ethical dilemmas. In addition three themes related to ethics are discussed: (1) Ethics is concerned with morality and ethical theory; (2) ethics encompasses reasoned thinking and moral justification; and (3) ethics requires a decision or action based on moral reasoning. Ethical dilemmas are then discussed in terms of conflicts they may engender. Finally, five strategies to facilitate the resolution of ethical dilemmas are outlined.

ETHICS

Ethics is a branch of philosophy that focuses on questions of right and wrong or good and evil in human character or conduct. Ethics encompasses both ethical theory and morality and is concerned with judgments about what one morally ought to do. Ethics has been defined as follows:

- Ethics is the study of rational processes for determining the best course of action in the face of conflicting [moral] choices. (Brody, 1981, p. 24)
- Ethics . . . [is] the systematic examination of the moral life [and] is designed to illuminate what we ought to do by asking us to consider and reconsider our ordinary actions, judgments, and justifications. (Beauchamp & Childress, 1983, p. xii)
- Ethics . . . is concerned with doing good and avoiding harm. (Bandman & Bandman, 1990)

- Ethics . . . is an attempt to formulate and justify systematic responses to the following question: "What, *all things considered,* ought to be done in a given situation?" (Benjamin & Curtis, 1986, p. 9)

Key themes within these definitions are: (1) Ethics is concerned with morality and ethical theory; (2) ethics encompasses reasoned thinking and moral justification; and (3) ethics requires a decision or action based on moral reasoning. A definition of ethics derived from these themes is as follows: Ethics is a systematic process of reflection in which issues of what one morally ought to do are analyzed, decided, and evaluated through moral reasoning that encompasses, but is not limited to, ethical principles and theories.

Ethics Is Concerned with Morality and Ethical Theory

What is morality, and what is its relationship to ethics? Morality refers to established and sanctioned rules of right and wrong that are culturally transmitted. Common examples are "one should keep promises," "one should not lie," and "one should not steal." Morality manifests itself through social institutions such as families, schools, and churches. Within these institutions right and wrong are taught, learned, and transmitted from generation to generation. Thus, the history of morality extends over the range of human experience and is not confined to philosophical contexts of ethics.

Ethics, however, is a subset of both morality and philosophy. Ethics encompasses ethical theory and is primarily philosophical and process oriented. It is concerned with rational, systematic, critical, and principled thinking regarding how one ought to live a moral life. The ethicist's job is to think clearly, thereby introducing lucidity, substance, and precision into reflection on morality. For example, in reflecting upon the moral rule that "one should keep promises," the ethicist might first clarify various definitions of promise keeping and then proceed to illuminate under what circumstances promises ought to be kept or broken.

Differences between morality and ethics have been noted by several authors. According to Thompson and Thompson (1985, pp. 4–5), morality consists of what a person ought to do in order to conform to acceptable social standards, whereas ethics consists of the philosophical reasons for and against the moral oughts or ought nots proposed by society. Jameton (1984, pp. 4–5) sees morality as the commitment of persons to follow values and principles operative in society, whereas he sees ethics as the systematic and philosophical study of values and principles. Beauchamp (1982, p. 6) views morality as "a social institution with a code of learnable rules" and ethics as systematic reflection upon the moral life. Despite these differences, however, the terms are often used interchangeably because of their interrelatedness. Morality gives substance to ethics, and ethics gives clarity and justification to morality through analysis and application of ethical principles and theory.

What, then, makes an action moral or ethical? Beauchamp (1982, pp. 11–14) identifies four characteristics associated with morality:

1. Morality overrides other human values;
2. Morality is concerned with prescriptive imperatives;
3. Morality is concerned with universalizability; and
4. Morality has an other-regarding focus.

Each of these is described in the following along with its limitations.

Morality Overrides Other Human Values. According to this thesis, certain rules, principles, and ideals have acquired moral status because of their overriding importance to individuals or to society. Rules such as "do not kill" or "do not steal" are considered overriding because they are essential to the moral functioning and stability of a society. Individuals or societies who endorse them give them priority over other values in life. For example, conscientious objectors who refuse to serve in the Armed Forces because they cannot kill accept "not killing" as their overriding action guide.

A problem with this thesis is that nonmoral events sometimes take overriding priority in our lives. In other words, moral conditions do not *always* (and some would say should not *always*) take precedence over other human values because sometimes moral rightness may seem less important than other considerations. For fear of a lawsuit, a nurse administrator may follow a legal course of action even when the nurse administrator feels that this may not be in the patient's best interest. Therefore some persons dispute whether overriding action guides are a necessary condition of morality.

Morality Is Concerned with Prescriptive Imperatives. This characteristic of morality focuses on the oughts and ought nots that guide human behavior by prescribing actions or restraints to actions. "One ought to tell the truth" or "one ought not to steal" are examples of prescriptive imperatives. Not all oughts and ought nots fall within the domain of morality, however. Rules of etiquette (e.g., "one ought to address a monsignor as The Right Reverend Monsignor") or rules of art (e.g., "one ought to use the edges of the paper to determine angles") are examples of oughts that fall outside the domain of morality. Therefore, morality is concerned with what one *morally* ought to do, not just with what one ought to do. As such, *moral* oughts and ought nots are concerned with right and wrong or good and evil.

Despite this emphasis, not all language with moral import can be translated into prescriptive imperatives. The statement that "Beth is a morally courageous woman" suggests a moral virtue, yet it is not a prescriptive imperative. Similarly, the statement that "Bob is a man of high integrity" suggests a moral virtue, yet it is not a prescriptive imperative. Virtues are character traits that dispose individuals to proper motivation and to do what is morally right or commendable, and therefore virtues are correctly associated with morality. Despite this association, however, virtues cannot easily be translated into prescriptive imperatives, thus highlighting a problem with such imperatives as a necessary characteristic of morality.

Another problem of prescriptive imperatives as a characteristic of morality relates to supererogatory acts. Supererogatory acts are those actions that go beyond the call of duty; that is, they exceed common moral standards. Although praiseworthy, supererogatory acts are optional, not matters of duty. Since moral prescriptions specify one's moral duties but do not go beyond them, these prescriptive imperatives do not accommodate supererogatory acts. To illustrate, suppose while driving home from work a nurse administrator sees an accident in which a young man is injured. The nurse stops, gives immediate care, and then uses CB Channel 9 to request emergency assistance. We would probably agree that the nurse administrator's duty is done. But further suppose that this person now stops at the nearest telephone booth and calls the wife of the injured man to alert her to the accident. We would probably agree that the nurse administrator has gone beyond duty. Prescriptive statements do not easily accommodate this type of supererogatory action. Consequently prescriptive language does not incorporate all of morality, for it not only eliminates virtues but also supererogatory actions.

Morality Is Concerned with Universalizability. According to this thesis, all similar persons in relevantly similar situations ought to be treated similarly. This notion, addressed by Singer (1961, p. 5) in his generalization principle, states that *"What is right (or wrong) for one person must be right (or wrong) for any similar person in similar circumstances."* The principle requires that whenever a particular act is judged as right or wrong, all relevantly similar acts must also be judged as right or wrong.

If withholding the truth about advanced cancer is deemed justifiable for Patient A, then it must also be deemed justifiable for Patient B, Patient C, and so forth *if* no relevant differences exist among these patients or their situations. If withholding the truth about advanced cancer is deemed justifiable for Patient A but *not* for Patients B, C, and so forth, then relevant differences between Patient A and Patients B, C, and so forth must be specified and justified.

Relevant differences could be related to age, intelligence, or mental health. For example, suppose one woman diagnosed with advanced breast cancer has a history of excellent coping skills whenever under severe stress, whereas another woman with the same diagnosis has a history of severe depression and attempted suicides whenever under severe stress. In this situation a different approach to truthfulness for each of these women might be morally justified. If no relevant differences exist between these two women with advanced breast cancer, then they both ought to be treated alike regarding the truth.

As with the preceding characteristics of morality, however, generalizability also has been criticized. What do crucial terms within Singer's generalization principle mean? Who are similar persons? What are similar circumstances? And what are relevant differences? In addition to this criticism, the meaning of generalizability also has been questioned. Some persons have interpreted generalizability to mean that the same moral principles apply to all persons regardless of circumstances. That is, one would always tell the truth to all patients with advanced cancer regardless of their age, intelligence, mental health, or other distinguishing characteristics. This interpretation of generalizability is considered by many philosophers to be simplistic for it does not accommodate personal choice or cultural differences.

Morality Has An Other-Regarding Focus. This characteristic of morality focuses on the welfare of others through actively benefiting or preventing harm to them. It differs from the preceding characteristics because of its focus on content (i.e., human welfare) rather than on structure (e.g., prescriptive imperatives). An other-regarding focus may take the form of showing compassion for a patient in pain, helping a student successfully complete a thesis, or preventing harm to a friend by forewarning the friend of some danger.

Although an other-regarding focus is appealing as a characteristic of morality, it contains ambiguities. For example, whose welfare is to be taken into consideration? Everyone's? The majority of persons? Persons most affected by a decision? What happens when ensuring the welfare of some persons unwittingly causes harm to other persons? Is disregard of self morally tenable? Questions such as these raise issues that need further clarification regarding this fourth characteristic of morality.

In summary, the preceding four characteristics suggest that morality may not be a single tidy concept but one composed of many strands. As no specific characteristic captures the complexity of morality, one should not place unyielding confidence in a single characteristic or set of characteristics. When each characteristic is added to the next, however, one's confidence in a circumstance being a moral situation increases. If all four characteristics of morality exist, then a situation involving morality most likely exists. Once we are reasonably sure that a situation involving morality exists, that situation most likely will demand our reasoned thinking and ability to justify a moral stand.

Ethics Encompasses Reasoned Thinking and Moral Justification

What is the focus of reasoned thinking in ethics? The focus is *moral* reasoning. This is a way of thinking in which a person's deliberations about what is morally right or morally wrong must be justified by appeals to moral reasons. These appeals provide independent grounds (i.e., grounds outside of oneself) for why others should agree that an act is morally right or morally wrong. In moral reasoning, no judgment made on moral grounds is immune from critical evaluation.

According to Beauchamp and Childress (1983, pp. 4–6), moral reasons can be arranged in a hierarchy that includes judgments, rules, principles, and theories. In moving from specific justifications to more abstract ones, a judgment can be justified in terms of a rule, which in turn can be justified in terms of a principle, which in turn can be justified in terms of a theory. The strongest justification is coverage at all four levels of the hierarchy. These concepts are depicted in Table 1–1.

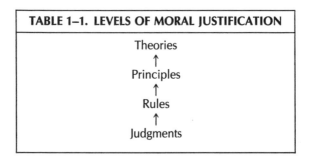

TABLE 1–1. LEVELS OF MORAL JUSTIFICATION
Theories
↑
Principles
↑
Rules
↑
Judgments

To further clarify these concepts, key terms are defined and then applied to a situation where a nurse administrator makes a decision not to admit additional seriously ill patients to an understaffed intensive care unit.

A **judgment,** when applied to moral justification, is a determination about rightness or wrongness based on a deliberative process. It is specific to a situation and may or may not have independent grounding because it is one person's judgment. For example, based on deliberation, a nurse administrator might determine not to admit additional seriously ill patients to an intensive care unit because there are too few registered nurses on the unit. This judgment may or may not have adequate justification.

A **rule,** when applied to moral justification, is a fixed guide for ethical conduct or action. It extends beyond a given situation and has more independent grounding that a judgment. A nurse administrator might justify not admitting additional seriously ill patients to an understaffed intensive care unit by applying the following rule: "In Hospital X, level of patient acuity and available staff to meet this acuity level are commensurate."

A **principle,** when applied to moral justification, is an abstract but fundamental guide for moral action that possesses generality and independent grounding. A nurse administrator might justify not admitting additional seriously ill patients to an understaffed nursing unit by applying the following principle of respect for persons.

Patients are human beings. Human beings possess intrinsic dignity and worth; therefore, they deserve respect. Since patients are human beings, they also deserve respect. To place patients in a situation of potential harm, as might occur on an understaffed intensive care unit, would show disregard for them as human beings, thus violating the principle of respect for persons.

Lastly, a **theory,** when applied to moral justification, is a set of interrelated moral principles and rules. A theory possesses both generality and independent grounding. A nurse administrator might justify not admitting additional seriously ill patients to an understaffed intensive care unit by applying the ethical theory of deontology. Deontology is a type of ethical theory in which features of acts other than, or in addition to, their consequences determine what makes an act right or wrong. (Chapter 2 focuses on ethical theories.) In the following excerpt, duty is the relevant right-making feature.

It is one's duty to show respect for patients as persons. Placing patients in situations of potential harm shows lack of respect for them, thus, violating one's duty. Therefore, the right act (i.e., the one that allows one's duty to be carried out) is not to admit additional seriously ill patients to an understaffed intensive care unit.

To summarize, a nursing judgment about what morally ought to be done with seriously ill patients in understaffed conditions was justified by a rule, which in turn was justified by a principle, which in turn was justified by a theory. The nurse administrator's responsibility, however, does not end just with not admitting additional seriously ill patients to a given unit. Seriously ill patients cannot be abandoned without care. The nurse administrator must either arrange for experienced nurses from another unit to oversee the patients' care or find additional help for the intensive care unit. These strategies require a decision and/or action.

Ethics Requires a Decision or Action Based on Moral Reasoning

The third theme identified in the definitions of ethics that began this chapter is that ethics requires a decision or action. We want to know what morally one ought to do. An approach staff nurses and nurse administrators have found helpful in such deliberations is use of a systematic problem-solving framework. Such a framework is described in depth in Chapter 5 but briefly outlined here to illustrate what the steps of such a framework might encompass.

Ethics Decision Framework

I. Data Collection and Assessment
   A. Situational Considerations
   B. Health Team Considerations
   C. Organizational Considerations

II. Problem Identification
   A. Ethical Considerations
   B. Nonethical Considerations
III. Consideration of Possible Actions
   A. Utilitarian Thinking
   B. Deontological Thinking
IV. Decision and Selection of Course of Action
   A. Contribution of Internal/Group Factors
   B. Contribution of External Factors
   C. Quality of Decision and Course of Action
V. Reflection on Decision and Course of Action
   A. Reflection on Decision
   B. Reflection on Course of Action

In review, based on the three preceding themes associated with ethics, we can define ethics as a systematic process of reflection in which issues of what one morally ought to do are analyzed, decided, and evaluated through moral reasoning that encompasses, but is not limited to, ethical principles and theories. This systematic process of reflection is useful for analyzing ethical dilemmas, a topic to which we now turn.

ETHICAL DILEMMAS

When something is amiss in our moral life, we feel tense, guilty, confused, angry, or pained. For at the heart of this amissness is a sense that something wrong is happening or about to happen. This amissness is compounded when we are in the middle of the situation and don't know what to do about it. Here we often encounter ethical dilemmas. The following definitions help us to see why they are so troublesome:

- Some evidence indicates that act X is morally right, and some evidence indicates that act X is morally wrong, but the evidence on both sides is inconclusive. Abortion, for example, is sometimes said to be "a terrible dilemma" for women who see the evidence in this way. (Beauchamp & Childress, 1983, p. 4)
- It is clear to the agent that, on moral grounds, he or she both ought and ought not to perform act X. For example, some have

viewed the intentional cessation of lifesaving therapies in the case of comatose patients as dilemmatic for this reason. (Beauchamp & Childress, 1983, p. 4)

Rephrased, an ethical dilemma is a puzzling moral problem in which one is faced with what ought to be done in the face of competing moral alternatives. Thus, ethical dilemmas necessarily involve some form of moral conflict.

Ethical Dilemmas Often Involve Moral Conflict

Ethical dilemmas often involve one or more of the following types of moral conflict. These conflicts have been adapted from the work of Smith and Davis (1980).

1. A conflict between ethical principles.
2. A conflict of evidence.
3. A conflict between unsatisfactory alternatives.
4. A conflict between role obligations and personal ethics.
5. A conflict between ethics and law.

Each of these conflicts is discussed, with examples given to highlight the conflict.

A Conflict Between Ethical Principles. If a nurse administrator responsible for managing programs for emotionally handicapped persons worries about underprotection versus overprotection of those persons, the administrator is in conflict. This conflict involves two ethical principles—the principle of nonmaleficence and the principle of respect for autonomy. If persons with emotional handicaps are given too much decision making freedom, they could be harmed because of their diminished judgment. This harm could violate the ethical principle of nonmaleficence, which can be stated as follows: Do no harm. If persons with emotional handicaps are given too little decision making freedom, however, they could be robbed of the dignity that arises from governing their own lives. This loss of dignity not only violates their self-respect but also the ethical principle of respect for autonomy, which can be stated as follows: Autonomous persons should be free to choose and to act without having controlling constraints placed on them by others. Whether the principle of nonmaleficence or respect for autonomy should take precedence in this situation is based on, for example: (1) the nature and degree of the emotional handicap, (2) the nature of the situation to which the principles apply, and (3) the value ascribed to each principle by persons involved in and responsible for the decision. (Chapter 3 focuses on ethical principles.)

A Conflict of Evidence. A timely example of this conflict relates to development of policies and procedures for nursing care of patients with acquired immunodeficiency syndrome (AIDS) (Cecchi, 1986). Scientists now know that the most likely cause of AIDS is the human immunodeficiency virus (HIV) and that AIDS is transmitted by sexual contact; by direct inoculation with contaminated syringes, needles, or blood products; and from mother to baby in utero and through breast-feeding (Bennett, 1986; Klug, 1986; Levine & Bermel, 1986). Much still remains unknown because the disease is relatively new to the United States, with the first cases appearing in 1978. Consequently, accurate evidence is hard to obtain, and conflicting evidence exists about how to care for AIDS patients and how best to protect staff and laboratory workers. This latter point was highlighted in an article appearing in *The Washington Post* (Hilts, 1988, January 4) that described how a National Institutes of Health laboratory worker became infected with the HIV virus despite apparently following the Centers for Disease Control guidelines. Therefore, the best course of action to take to protect staff and laboratory workers from patients with HIV and to protect AIDS patients (with their compromised immune system) from staff remains difficult to resolve.

A Conflict Between Unsatisfactory Alternatives. An example that involves unsatisfactory alternatives is the predicament of Elizabeth Bouvia (Annas, 1984; Kane, 1985). Ms Bouvia is the young woman who wanted the courts to mandate the cooperation of a California hospital in her planned suicide by starvation. Cerebral palsy has left Ms Bouvia with no motor functioning except for minimal control of her right hand. When Ms Bouvia refused to eat at the hospital, the chief of psychiatry there testified that he would force feed her with a nasogastric tube if necessary. In a court decision made on December 16, 1983, Judge John H. Hews found Ms Bouvia fully competent to make decisions about her life. Nevertheless, the judge ruled in favor of forced feedings because of the devastating effects he anticipated that a patient starving herself to death would have on hospital personnel and on other physically handicapped persons in similar situations throughout the country. This was clearly a situation with unsatisfactory alternatives: If Ms Bouvia did not eat, death would occur, but if Ms Bouvia were force fed, respect for her personal autonomy would be severely violated.

According to Annas (1986), in 1984 Ms Bouvia fled to Mexico in an unsuccessful attempt to seek her death. She then returned to the

United States where she was a model patient at two facilities; however, on December 23, 1985, she was transferred again. At the new facility she had been eating modestly, but physicians determined her intake was insufficient for adequate rehabilitation and again began to force feed her. Another lawsuit to discontinue the nasogastric feeding tube was filed but denied by the judge, as the judge believed Ms Bouvia was still trying to starve herself to death. This opinion is on appeal, and the conflict between unsatisfactory alternatives continues.

A Conflict Between Role Obligations and Personal Ethics. Sometimes the ethical principles that nurses personally uphold conflict with their job expectations. A common example is that of the nurse who is asked to participate in an abortion as part of his or her job but feels that abortions violate the ethical principle of respect for persons. Obviously this nurse views a fetus as a person in contrast to other nurses who may not hold this view. Another example of this conflict is the one discussed by Smith and Davis (1980) in which a patient admitted for surgery is also on a methadone maintenance program. As part of the nurse's role in giving care, the nurse is expected to give the patient methadone. The nurse, however, views methadone programs as unethical because they harm patients by keeping them in a state of drug dependency. In both situations the nurse must decide whether to give the expected, role-obligated nursing care or to refuse the assignment and, thereby, uphold personal ethical principles. Despite the strength of the nurse's personal convictions, the nurse must understand that role expectations also incur strong moral obligations. Moral obligations inherent in role expectations may even take precedence over one's personal ethics. Nurses have strong moral role obligations not to abandon patients in their care without due cause and without ensuring their proper care.

A Conflict Between Ethics and Law. If one believes that morality always overrides other considerations, then this conflict between ethics and law does not exist. If one does not ascribe to the supremacy condition of morality, however, then potential conflicts between law and ethics may arise.

Although the desired (and usual) state of affairs is that ethics and law are congruent (i.e., that which is ethical is also legal; that which is unethical is also illegal), this condition does not always occur. Discrepancies in this relationship can take the following forms: (1) an action is ethical but illegal (e.g., some would say euthanasia); or (2) an action is unethical but legal (e.g., some would say abortion). Therefore, unless one is prepared to embark upon a course of civil disobedience, the final resolution of an ethical issue may depend upon legal considerations. Nevertheless, although legal considerations may affect ethical decisions, legal considerations are *not* intrinsic to ethical decisions and, thus, they should not be confused with right or wrong (Curtin, 1982a, p. 61). Understanding the relationship between law and ethics is important because legal considerations too often immobilize nurse administrators from thinking seriously about the rightness and wrongness of actions. Too often, when dealing with an ethical dilemma, the first question raised is: "Is it legal to do X?" If one is dealing with an ethical dilemma, however, the more important question to ask is: "Is it ethical to do X?"

In summary, then, ethical dilemmas are puzzling moral problems about what ought to be done in the face of competing moral choices. By identifying types of moral conflict, the nature of the tension within a moral conflict is clarified, thus helping to make the dilemma more manageable. In the following section, other strategies for making an ethical dilemma more manageable are discussed.

Ethical Dilemmas Are Often Manageable

Although ethical dilemmas may be complex, they are often manageable. Manageable does not necessarily mean that a tidy, happy, or comfortable solution will be found. Rather, it means that through use of moral reasoning and application of relevant facts, one can reduce an ethical dilemma into its component parts, making it more understandable and less puzzling. As a result a morally justified course of action can be initiated that helps mitigate the dilemma.

To facilitate the management of ethical dilemmas, Beauchamp (1982, pp. 52–56) offers five common sense strategies:

1. Obtain critical facts revelant to the moral controversy.
2. Reach agreement on definition of terms.
3. Reach agreement on a common framework of moral principles.
4. Use examples and counterexamples.
5. Expose the problems inherent in a line of reasoning.

Each of these strategies is discussed in the following in detail, with examples given.

Obtain Critical Facts Relevant to the Moral Controversy. Obtaining critical facts is important because decisions about moral matters often turn on the basis of facts. For example, to assess whether harm could come to nurses caring for AIDS patients requires accurate facts about

how AIDS is transmitted. In September 1986, Bennett summarized
what is known about AIDS transmission.

Current Factual Information on Transmission of AIDS[1]

Passing It On. HIV [human immunodeficiency virus] is transmitted
by sexual contact; by direct inoculation with contaminated blood
products, needles or syringes; and from mother to newborn in utero
and through breastfeeding. Transmission is dose-related. Despite the
fact that low concentrations of virus are sometimes present in saliva,
tears, urine, sweat and other body fluids, nonsexual household
transmission does not occur even when living conditions are
crowded, when eating utensils are shared or during hugging and
kissing.

Exposure occurs when blood or semen that contain infected
lymphocytes get into an uninfected person's bloodstream. Safe sex
practices can eliminate exposure: using a condom; refraining from
activities that can injure mucous membranes or impair skin integrity;
and not allowing body fluids—especially semen and blood—from
one partner to enter the other.

Sexual activities that do not involve the exchange or passing
of any body fluids between partners are considered safe.

Since the skin is an effective barrier, concern about
nonsexual exposure is only for invasive procedures and situations
where the skin is not intact.

Based on these facts, it would be morally indefensible for a nurse
with intact skin to refuse to feed or ambulate an AIDS patient; however, there would be justification to protect a nurse with skin lesions
from HIV while the nurse was handling blood or a contaminated nee-
dle from an AIDS patient.

---

[1]From: Bennett, J. A. (1986). AIDS beyond the hospital: A two-part CE feature. What we
know about AIDS. *American Journal of Nursing, 86,* 1016–1021.

Reach Agreement on Definition of Terms. If persons responsible for managing an ethical dilemma define key terms differently, resolution of the dilemma will be difficult. In discussing euthanasia, for example, Curtin (1982b, pp. 219–238) offers 15 definitions of this term based on different categories including: (1) voluntary mercy killing, (2) involuntary mercy killing, (3) voluntary withholding of treatment, and (4) involuntary withholding of treatment. These four terms are defined to point out how lack of a common definition can cause communication problems.

Voluntary mercy killing. This is the direct killing of an individual per that individual's request. More specifically it implies the killing of a hopelessly sick or injured person in a relatively painless way for reasons of mercy. For example, a husband gives his wife a lethal dose of morphine per her request in order to end her intolerable suffering from terminal cancer.

Involuntary mercy killing. This is the direct killing of an individual for reasons of mercy but without the individual's consent or without proxy consent. An obstetrician, for example, suffocates a severely acephalous newborn with multiple life-threatening and grotesque birth defects.

Voluntary withholding of treatment. A patient who knows that death is imminent without a certain treatment freely opts to reject such treatment although this patient clearly understands the benefits and risks. In one case a friend of the author's, in her forties, freely chose no medical or surgical interventions for breast cancer.

Involuntary withholding of treatment. Treatment that offers little hope of success is withheld from a person without the person's consent, although the person was capable of giving consent. For example, a wife does not tell her alert husband of an experimental treatment that could prolong his life for a few weeks because the cost of the treatment is so expensive that it would wipe out their modest life savings.

As these definitions show, until persons involved in ethical dilemmas reach a workable agreement on the definition of terms, they will have difficulty moving forward in the resolution of the dilemmas.

Reach Agreement on a Common Framework of Moral Principles. Since principles are fundamental guides to actions, they help us make decisions. If in confronting an ethical dilemma, however, some persons use one set of principles and other persons use a different set, management of the dilemma may be difficult. By discussing moral principles that seem to bear on an ethical dilemma and by seeking out the commonalities of these principles, a common framework may be found.

For instance, two nurse administrators strongly disagree over the issue of whether or not their staff nurses should participate in a citywide nurses' strike. Nurse Administrator A argues that the long-term consequences of the strike will benefit all persons involved (i.e., both patients and the nursing staff) and, therefore, the nurses are morally justified in striking. Nurse Administrator B argues that the strike makes patients pawns of the system, and therefore, the nurses are morally obligated *not* to strike. The basis of Nurse Administrator A's argument is the principle of utility (an action or practice is right, when compared with any other action or practice, if it leads to the greatest possible balance of good consequences, or to the least possible balance of bad consequences, for all persons affected by the action or practice); the basis of Nurse Administrator B's argument is the principle of respect for persons (to respect another person means to treat that person as an end and never as a mere means to an end). When both nurse administrators understand that they share the common goal of quality patient care (based on the ethical principle of beneficence), then they are able to resolve their differences.

Use Examples and Counterexamples. This strategy, common to law and debate, uses examples to make a point and counterexamples to dispute the point. To illustrate, one nurse administrator strongly supports telling the truth to seriously ill cancer patients in all circumstances based on examples from personal experience, whereas another nurse administrator disputes this position based on counterexamples also taken from personal experience. A sample dialogue follows.

EXAMPLE: **Nurse Administrator A:** In my ten years of experience as a nurse administrator on an oncology unit, I have talked with several hundred patients with cancer. They tell me they want to know the truth about their diagnosis and treatment. It makes them feel in control of their lives. I agree with them.
COUNTEREXAMPLE: **Nurse Administrator B:** I, too, have had considerable experience talking with cancer patients over the years. While what you say is true for most of these patients, it is not true for all of them. I have seen several instances where patients who insisted they wanted to know the truth about their diagnosis could not cope with it when they heard it. They became severely

depressed and lost their will to live. Unfortunately two of these patients with a long and painful family history of cancer committed suicide.

After more discussion of these points, using examples and counterexamples, the nurse administrators agreed that while, overall, it was desirable to tell the truth to patients with cancer, there were some circumstances where it would be morally justifiable to postpone the truth or deny it.

Expose the Problems Inherent in a Line of Reasoning. When the strategy of critical analysis is applied to ethical dilemmas, it means that one is attuned to any inconsistencies, gaps, irrelevancies, or errors in one's own or other's moral reasoning. If such flaws exist, then the argument for a certain moral position may need to be modified so that the argument becomes more defensible. To illustrate, a sample dialogue follows.

Nurse Administrator A: You say you strongly believe that Mr. Jones has a right to refuse surgery and that you will support his decision.
Nurse Administrator B: Yes, that is my position. I believe patients have a right to make decisions that affect their lives, even if we don't agree with them.
Nurse Administrator A: Do you feel there are any exceptions to your position?
Nurse Administrator B: Yes, if the patient is going to harm another person.
Nurse Administrator A: But what if the patient harms another person in self-defense?
Nurse Administrator B: I would then need to clarify my position to say: "I would restrict a patient's liberty if the patient harmed another person *without due cause.*"
Nurse Administrator A: Do you believe that if the patient harmed himself because of his decision that you should restrict his liberty?
Nurse Administrator B: No.
Nurse Administrator A: But what if the patient is under the influence of heavy sedation or is severely depressed when he makes the decision?

Nurse Administrator B: I hadn't considered those possibilities, but, on reflection, I think it might be proper to restrict the liberty of a patient with these problems. Mr. Jones, however, has none of these problems. He is well informed about the surgery and the pros and cons of the surgery. He is of sound mind, and his decision to refuse the surgery is his own. Therefore, I still support my position in regard to Mr. Jones, but I would modify my position in other circumstances where limiting a person's liberty seemed morally defensible.

Individually or taken as a group, these five strategies facilitate deliberation about ethical dilemmas. Although these strategies may not always resolve the dilemma, they help nurse administrators to become clearer about the nature and management of the dilemma.

Summary. In this chapter, the terms *ethics* and *ethical dilemmas* are defined. *Ethics* is a systematic process of reflection in which issues of what one morally ought to do are analyzed, decided, and evaluated through moral reasoning that encompasses, but is not limited to, ethical principles and theories. *Ethical dilemmas* are puzzling moral problems in which one is faced with what ought to be done in the face of competing moral choices. Ethical dilemmas often involve conflict, for example, a conflict between ethical principles or a conflict between role obligations and personal ethics. The management of ethical dilemmas can be clarified through use of facts, common terminology, common frameworks, examples and counterexamples, and critical analysis of moral arguments. With ethics and ethical dilemmas now defined, the nurse administrator is in a better position to understand the classical ethical theories presented in Chapter 2.

REFERENCES

Annas, G. J. (1984). When suicide prevention becomes brutality: The case of Elizabeth Bouvia. *The Hastings Center Report*, 14(2), 20–21, 46.

Annas, G. J. (1986). At law—Elizabeth Bouvia: Whose space is this anyway? *Hastings Center Report, 16*(2), 24–25.

Bandman, E. L., & Bandman, B. (1990). *Nursing ethics through the life span* (2nd ed.). Norwalk, CT: Appleton & Lange.

Beauchamp, T. L. (1982). *Philosophical ethics: An introduction to moral philosophy.* New York: McGraw–Hill.

Beauchamp, T. L., & Childress, J. F. (1983). *Principles of biomedical ethics* (2nd ed.). New York: Oxford University Press.

Benjamin, M., & Curtis, J. (1986). *Ethics in nursing* (2nd ed.). New York: Oxford University Press.

Bennett, J. A. (1986). AIDS beyond the hospital: A two-part CE feature. What we know about AIDS. *American Journal of Nursing, 86,* 1016–1021.

Brody, H. (1981). *Ethical decisions in medicine* (2nd ed.). Boston: Little, Brown.

Cecchi, R. (1986). Living with AIDS: When the system fails. *American Journal of Nursing, 86,* 45–47.

Curtin, L. (1982a). No rush to judgment. In L. Curtin & M. J. Flaherty, *Nursing ethics: Theories and pragmatics* (pp. 57–63). Bowie, MD: Brady.

Curtin, L. (1982b). Case study IV: Consent, conflict, and "euthanasia." In L. Curtin & M. J. Flaherty, *Nursing ethics: Theories and pragmatics* (pp. 219–238). Bowie, MD: Brady.

Hilts, P. J. (1988, January 4). AIDS in the lab: Questions of safety. *The Washington Post,* p. A11.

Jameton, A. (1984). *Nursing practice: The ethical issues.* Englewood Cliffs, NJ: Prentice Hall.

Kane, F. I. (1985). Keeping Elizabeth Bouvia alive for the public good. *Hastings Center Report, 15*(6), 5–8.

Klug, R. M. (1986). AIDS beyond the hospital: Part two of a CE feature. Children with AIDS. *American Journal of Nursing, 86,* 1126–1132.

Levine, C., & Bermel, J. (Eds.). (1986). AIDS: Public health and civil liberties [Special supplement]. *Hastings Center Report, 16*(6), 1–36.

Singer, M. G. (1961). *Generalization in ethics: An essay in the logic of ethics, with the rudiments of a system of moral philosophy.* New York: Knopf.

Smith, S. J., & Davis, A. J. (1980). Ethical dilemmas: Conflicts among rights, duties, and obligations. *American Journal of Nursing, 80,* 1462–1466.

Thompson, J. E., & Thompson, H. O. (1985). *Bioethical decision making for nurses.* Norwalk, CT: Appleton–Century–Crofts.

2

Classical Ethical Theories

Mary Cipriano Silva

Experience without theory is blind
but theory without experience
is mere intellectual play.
Immanuel Kant

In this chapter the basics of two classical ethical theories are presented: utilitarianism and deontology. For each of these theories the following are discussed: underlying principle(s), types, and criticisms and defenses. In addition, a mixed ethical theory is introduced to show how aspects of both utilitarianism and deontology can be combined into a viable alternative to pure utilitarianism or deontology.

Underlying every moral judgment are implicit assumptions about rightness and wrongness. Too often, however, these assumptions have not been thought through or formalized into an explicit ethical framework. We make moral decisions but are unsure of how we arrive at or might justify them. The purpose of this chapter is to make this path seem less uncertain by discussing justification by appeal to ethical theories.

In any discipline knowledge changes over time. Nevertheless, there are works of such excellence and influence that they endure. These classics serve as standards for testing new ideas or reformulating old ones. Classical philosophical writings on utilitarianism are frequently associated with John Stuart Mill (1806–1873); classical philosophical writings on deontology are frequently associated with Immanuel Kant (1724–1804). Because subsequent philosophical refinements of both utilitarianism and deontology are based on the writings of these two philosophers, their writings are emphasized in this chapter.

CLASSICAL UTILITARIAN THEORY

Underlying Principle: The Principle of Utility

As formulated by John Stuart Mill, the following excerpt on the principle of utility is a succinct summary of utilitarianism. The summary does not include the entirety of Mill's development of the topic; however, it does highlight some important points.

John Stuart Mill on The Principle of Utility[1]

The creed which accepts as the foundation of morals "utility" or the "greatest happiness principle" holds that *actions are right in proportion as they tend to promote happiness; wrong as they tend to produce the reverse of happiness* [italics added]. By happiness is intended pleasure and the absence of pain; by unhappiness, pain and the privation of pleasure. To give a clear view of the moral standard set up by the theory, much more requires to be said; in particular, what things it includes in the ideas of pain and pleasure, and to what extent this is left an open question. But these supplementary explanations do not affect the theory of life on which this theory of morality is grounded— namely, *that pleasure and freedom from pain are the only things desirable as ends* [italics added]; and that all desirable things (which are as numerous in the utilitarian as in any other scheme) are desirable either for pleasure inherent in themselves or as a means to the promotion of pleasure and the prevention of pain. (p. 7)

Based on the preceding definition, what are the essential characteristics of the principle of utility? First, the rightness or wrongness of an act depends on the consequences produced by the act. Second, the consequences produced by an act may cause either happiness (pleasure and the absence of pain) or unhappiness (privation of pleasure and the presence of pain). Thus, utilitarianism is essentially a trade-off philoso-

---

[1]**From:** Mill, J. S. (1979). *Utilitarianism* (G. Sher, Ed.). Indianapolis: Hackett. (Original work published 1861) Reprinted by permission of Hackett Publishing Co., Inc., Indianapolis, Indiana.

phy: one that maximizes good and minimizes harm in trade-off situations. Lastly, those acts whose consequences promote happiness tend to be right actions, whereas those acts whose consequences promote unhappiness tend to be wrong actions. The utilitarian notion of consequences as the determining factor of rightness or wrongness is important because it rules out other criteria for rightness or wrongness such as the intrinsic nature of the act itself. As a result, in utilitarianism no act is right or wrong outside of the consequences (Brody & Engelhardt, 1987, pp. 3–4).

But what consequences are desirable? According to Mill, the desired consequences are happiness or pleasure (terms he takes to be synonymous). Other philosophers sometimes disagree and consider health, knowledge, beauty, love, and friendship to be desired consequences independent of happiness or pleasure. Although it is beyond the scope of this book to pursue these disputes, it is within its scope to identify commonalities among utilitarians even when they differ. The first commonality is this: Desired consequences represent *intrinsic* values, whether they be health or happiness or truth or beauty. Put another way, the rightness of an act is partly determined by the intrinsic value of its consequences.

What does this mean? Intrinsic means belonging to or derived from the essential nature of a thing. In utilitarianism, intrinsic values are those values that are good in themselves and not as a means to something else. To illustrate, good health is an intrinsic value to some persons as opposed to food or exercise, which are necessary (although not necessarily sufficient) means to good health. Therefore, within utilitarianism good health would be a desired consequence for those persons holding it as an intrinsic value.

A second commonality shared by philosophers who hold utilitarian views is this: When assessing consequences, one looks at the effect of the consequences on *all those affected by the act or, according to some, on those most affected by the act.* In Mill's (1861/1979) words:

> I must again repeat what the assailants of utilitarianism seldom have the justice to acknowledge, that the happiness which forms the utilitarian standard of what is right in conduct is not the agent's own happiness but that of all concerned. As between his own happiness and that of others, utilitarianism requires him to be as strictly impartial as a disinterested and benevolent spectator. (p. 16) (Reprinted by permission of Hackett Publishing Co., Inc., Indianapolis, Indiana.)

In utilitarianism, one is balancing consequences to promote the greatest happiness; therefore, a decision-making approach similar to the following can be used:

1. Identify viable alternatives of an action.
2. Determine the consequences of each alternative.
3. From the predicted consequences, determine the intrinsic value and disvalue for each consequence.
4. Compare the net pleasure and pain for each alternative act.
5. Choose the act that produces the most net pleasure minus pain for all persons affected by, or most affected by, the act.

Types of Utilitarianism

There are two types of utilitarianism: act and rule. The difference focuses on whether the principle of utility is to be applied to specific acts in specific situations or to rules of conduct that determine the rightness or wrongness of an act. This conflict between specific acts and rules is a major ethical controversy in the mid-twentieth century (Veatch & Fry, 1987, p. 10).

Act Utilitarianism. In act utilitarianism appeals are made directly to the principle of utility to determine what is right or obligatory. If rules are used in act utilitarianism, they serve only as rules of thumb that can be broken if a situation demands it. The act utilitarian asks, "'What effect will *my* doing *this* act in *this* situation have on the general balance of good over evil?', not 'What effect will *everyone's* doing this *kind* of act in this *kind* of situation have on the general balance of good over evil?'" (Frankena, 1973, p. 35). The emphasis is on the greatest general good in a particular situation, even if in that particular situation a general moral rule such as telling the truth must be violated. Put another way, "It can never be right to act on the rule of telling the truth if we have good independent grounds for thinking that it would be for the greatest good not to tell the truth in a particular case" (Frankena, 1973, pp. 35–36).

Strengths of act utilitarianism include its sensitivity to particular cases and its recognition that abiding by a rule may violate the principle of utility because the greatest good for the greatest number may not be served. It is not too difficult to conceive of a situation where following a moral rule such as telling the truth could cause considerable harm and minimal good to persons affected by the situation. Thus abiding by a moral rule may violate the principle of utility.

A major problem with act utilitarianism, however, is that sometimes the decisions reached are morally wrong. This could occur when, for example, a specific act in a specific situation involves the breaking of a moral rule such as promise keeping. On act utilitarian grounds this rule would not need to be honored if, on balance, the breaking of the promise would cause more good than evil consequences to persons affected by this act in a particular situation. Nevertheless, on non-act-utilitarian grounds there are justifiable moral reasons for keeping promises: Commitments should be honored to ensure trust.

Rule Utilitarianism. In contrast to act utilitarianism is rule utilitarianism, where moral rules are important because of their significance to society. We first determine what rules (instead of what acts) produce the greatest utility. The principle of utility, therefore, serves as the standard by which rules are selected or discarded. According to Frankena (1973, p. 39), the rule utilitarian follows a rule because following the rule results in the greatest good for the greatest number. Put another way, in rule utilitarianism an act is right if it conforms to a moral rule that has been validated by the principle of utility.

Strengths of rule utilitarianism include its sensitivity to societal norms and its commitment to maximizing the greatest good for the greatest number. The sensitivity to societal norms helps to ensure that the rules that govern a society are not dominated by the whims of the few. The commitment to maximizing the greatest good for the greatest number helps to ensure that the best interests of the majority are protected.

As with act utilitarianism, rule utilitarianism also has some problems. The first problem focuses on the conflict of what ought to be done when a moral rule and the principle of utility conflict. For example, what does one do when telling the truth decreases, rather than increases, happiness or pleasure? Does one abide by the rule or does one abide by the principle of utility? The rule utilitarian view is that one abides by the rule because of the overall significance of obeying the rules, which express the basic terms of social agreement.

A second problem pertinent to rule utilitarianism can be addressed by two questions: (1) do all rules carry the same weight; and (2) what course of action does one take when there is a conflict between equally weighted rules? Regarding the first question, the response is that not all rules necessarily carry the same weight. Those rules that enhance utility more carry greater weight than those rules that enhance utility less. For instance, rules that deal with not harming patients frequently take precedence over rules that deal with patient preferences because the former increases utility more than the latter. Regarding the second question on a conflict of rules, the response is that utilitarianism does not demand one single right action. If in regard to an act, two (or more) equally weighted rules generate equal amounts of utility, then there are two (or possibly more) right courses of action.

In addition there is a third problem with moral rules—the problem of the extent of their generalizability. Ought a moral rule apply to all persons regardless of circumstances? Should the truth always be told regardless of age, culture, setting, physical and mental states, and so forth? As noted in Chapter 1, few persons would answer "yes" to this question because they do *not* interpret generalizability to mean that what is right or wrong for one person must be right or wrong for all other persons regardless of circumstances. Rather, the principle of generalizability most often is interpreted to mean that relevantly similar persons in relevantly similar situations have similar moral obligations. For example, if two persons have been so seriously injured that their judgments and emotions are profoundly and similarly impaired, then withholding a similar truth (death of a spouse or parent) may be morally justified by a physician or nurse. This position represents a compromise between treating every person or situation differently and treating every person or situation alike. A rule is being used, but it is a rule with a built-in qualifier—that persons who are more alike than unlike on relevant characteristics should be treated in a morally similar way.

Criticisms and Defenses of Utilitarianism

To put utilitarianism into perspective, let us examine how contemporary philosophers have both criticized and defended it. According to Beauchamp (1982, pp. 97–104), criticisms have included: (1) the problem of quantifying goodness, (2) the problem of unjust distributions, and (3) the problem of requiring supererogatory acts.

The Problem of Quantifying Goodness. Since utilitarians assess the value of consequences, the issue of measurement invariably arises. How does one measure the utility of intrinsic values such as happiness, truth, or friendship? How does one measure which of two competing intrinsic values maximizes utility and, thus, goodness? These questions raise issues about what can be measured (goods? values?) and how this measurement should occur (quantitatively? qualitatively?).

In defense of these concerns, utilitarians would agree that utilitarianism does require an assessment of values in terms of utility; however, it does not require a precision beyond one's capabilities. What it does require is an attempt to maximize utility through careful reasoning.

The Problem of Unjust Distributions. The problem concerns injustices that could occur to a minority if the utilitarian principle alone was followed. It concerns the loss of individual rights in the interests of the majority, leading to an unfair distribution of utility. An example of this type of conflict occurred in Beverly Hills, Calif. when the city banned smoking in most restaurants, retail stores, and public meetings (Mathews, 1987, February 19). Based on a U.S. surgeon general's report, the ban was justified on the grounds that passive inhaling of smoke is dangerous to one's health. Therefore, to protect the health interests of the majority in Beverly Hills, smoking was banned. Not all restaurateurs or other community members agreed with this position, maintaining that the ban was unfair because it violated their personal liberties.

Utilitarians would counter this criticism as follows: (1) Utilitarianism not only focuses on maximizing benefits but also on minimizing harms; and (2) rule utilitarianism takes into account moral rules of justice. Therefore one could argue that if maximizing benefits also causes an imbalanced or unproportional set of harms, then this stance would be unacceptable to a utilitarian because it violates the principle of utility. A stance more compatible with utilitarianism would be the establishment of an upper limit of tolerable harm, even if maximizing benefits would suffer. This upper limit of tolerable harm could be determined by appeals to rules of justice that are incompatible with unjustified harms to a minority group. The rules of justice, according to rule utilitarians, can be derived from appeal to the rule of utility.

The Problem of Requiring Supererogatory Acts. Utilitarianism also has been faulted for its inability to distinguish clearly between morally obligatory acts (those acts demanded by moral duty) and supererogatory acts (those acts beyond the demands of moral duty). This fault is of concern because if a clear distinction cannot be made between morally obligatory acts and morally optional acts, then utilitarianism as a theory may be too broad and demanding. As a result, utilitarians (in honoring the principle of utility) may be forced to adopt rules that exceed conventional social morality and, thus, also exceed most people's willingness to honor such rules.

In defense of these concerns, utilitarians argue that rules should not be established indiscriminately; that is, there should not be too many rules, too few rules, or rules with too many exceptions. According to Beauchamp (1982, p. 103), "Since moral rules restrict human freedom, the social value derived from the having of a rule must be greater than the value of the freedom that would be gained by not having the rule." Supererogatory acts that are required or too many rules could lead to disutility rather than utility because of the uncertainty and distrust they may cause. Nevertheless, supererogatory acts could be justified in extreme circumstances if more utility than disutility occurs (e.g., a private citizen willingly sacrifices his or her life to prevent the death of a U.S. president).

In summary, the following can be said about utilitarianism.

- Utilitarianism is a moral theory whose proponents endorse the premise that no acts are right or wrong outside of the consequences produced by the acts, and we often must trade off desirable results and undesirable results to obtain our goals.

- Desired consequences are those consequences that maximize intrinsic value for all persons affected or most affected by the act; undesirable consequences are those consequences that diminish intrinsic value for all persons affected or most affected by the act.
- The right act (i.e., the one that we are morally obligated to follow) is the one whose consequences produce the highest net balance of what is intrinsically good (e.g., pleasure, love, knowledge) minus what is intrinsically bad (e.g., illness, pain, or ignorance) for all persons affected or most affected by the act. This thesis is known as the principle of utility.
- There are two types of utilitarianism. In act utilitarianism specific acts in specific situations are viewed as unique, and the principle of utility is applied directly to each act. In rule utilitarianism moral rules intervene between an act and the principle of utility so that the principle of utility is applied to the rule and not to the individual act.
- Problems associated with utilitarianism include the problem of quantifying goodness, the problem of unjust distributions, and the problem of requiring supererogatory acts.

CLASSICAL DEONTOLOGICAL THEORY

Underlying Principle: The Categorical Imperative

With the underlying principle and types of classical utilitarian theory now defined, it is time to focus our attention on a second classical ethical theory: deontology. The purist form of classical deontological theory is represented herein by the writings of Immanuel Kant. The reader must keep in mind, however, that Kant's views represent a rather extreme type of deontology and that more moderate views exist. A more moderate view can be found in the work of W. D. Ross and is discussed later in this chapter. With these points in mind, the underlying principle and types of deontology are first defined; next, criticisms and defenses of it are summarized.

As formulated by Immanuel Kant, the underlying principle of deontology is the categorical imperative. The following excerpt is a succinct summary of the deontological perspective and does not show the entirety of Kant's development of this complex topic. Nevertheless, the excerpt describes background information leading up to the conceptualization of the categorical imperative, as well as one of Kant's formulations of it.

Immanuel Kant on
The Categorical Imperative[2]

There is no possibility of thinking of anything at all in the world, or
even out of it, which can be regarded as good without qualification,
except a *good will*. Intelligence, wit, judgment, and whatever talents
of the mind one might want to name are doubtless in many respects
good and desirable, as are such qualities of temperament as courage,
resolution, perseverance. But they can also become extremely bad
and harmful if the will, which is to make use of these gifts of nature
and which in its special constitution is called character, is not
good. . . . (p. 7)

The concept of a will estimable in itself and good without
regard to any further end must now be developed. This concept
already dwells in the natural sound understanding and needs not so
much to be taught as merely to be elucidated. It always holds first
place in estimating the total worth of our actions and constitutes the
condition of all the rest. Therefore, we shall take up the concept of
duty, which includes that of a good will, though with certain
subjective restrictions and hindrances, which far from hiding a good
will or rendering it unrecognizable, rather bring it out by contrast
and make it shine forth more brightly. . . . (p. 9)

If then there is to be a supreme practical principle and, as
far as the human will is concerned, a categorical imperative, then it
must be such that from the conception of what is necessarily an end
for everyone because this end is an end in itself it constitutes an
objective principle of the will and can hence serve as a practical law.
The ground of such a principle is this: rational nature exists as an
end in itself. In this way man necessarily thinks of his own existence;
thus far is it a subjective principle of human actions. But in this way
also does every other rational being think of his existence on the
same rational ground that holds also for me; . . . hence it is at the
same time an objective principle, from which, as a supreme practical
ground, all laws of the will must be able to be derived. The practical
imperative will therefore be the following: *Act in such a way that you
treat humanity, whether in your own person or in the person of another,
always at the same time as an end and never simply as a means* [italics
added]. (p. 36)

[2]**From:** Kant, I. (1981). *Grounding for the metaphysics of morals* (J. W. Ellington, Trans.).
Indianapolis: Hackett. (Original work published in German in 1785) Reprinted by permission of Hackett Publishing Co., Inc., Indianapolis, Indiana.

Based on the preceding, what are essentials of Kant's ethical theory? First, persons must act out of a good will. Second, acting from duty is central to a good will and morality. Third, persons should be treated as ends in themselves and never as mere means to the ends of others.

Let us now examine these concepts more precisely. According to Kant, a good will is one that is uncompromising in its motivation to do the right thing (i.e., duty) because it *is* the right thing. It is a will that knows what to do without reference to consequences. In its most conservative Kantian form, deontology (which comes from the Greek word *deon* meaning binding duty) is an ethical theory that is grounded in the following premise: An act is right only when it is done for the sake of duty.

In addition, the Kantian premise that persons should be treated as ends and never as mere means to ends is embodied in the categorical imperative. This imperative demands that every human be treated with dignity and worth because every human has an inherent worth equal to that of every other human. The dignity and worth of humans arise from their possession of rationality. Rationality confers dignity and worth upon humans because it recognizes their self-determining abilities. Rationality also allows humans to understand the implications of the categorical imperative; that is, a rational human would understand why the principle underlying the categorical imperative must be followed. To illustrate this point, Ellington (1981) explains:

> According to the formula of universal law, any violation of the formula of the end in itself must be wrong, i.e., when someone is treated as a mere means, his purposes are regarded as not counting; when the maxim of such treatment is universalized, the agent of such treatment must be willing to be so treated in turn. But here is a contradiction, for no one wants his purposes to count for nothing. Conversely, any violation of the formula of universal law always involves making oneself an exception to the rules (as when one lies). By doing so, he makes the aims of others mere means to his own selfish aims—he exploits others thereby, and the formula of the end in itself forbids such exploitation. Consequently, according to the formula of the end in itself, *any* [italics added] violation of the formula of universal law must be wrong. (p. x)

Thus, the preceding moral implication of the categorical imperative addresses generalizability and fairness. There can be no moral double standard—one standard for oneself and one standard for others. A double standard violates generalizability and diminishes the intrinsic value of all persons affected by it. In summary, then, the categorical imperative deals with two moral themes: (1) respect for persons as ends in themselves and (2) the principle of generalizability.

As previously noted, not all deontologists hold as conservative a view as did Kant. According to Beauchamp and Childress (1983, p. 33), some moderate deontologists ascribe to the following premise: Deontology is an ethical theory in which features of acts other than, or in addition to, their consequences make them right or wrong. What features? These features could be, but are not limited to, duties, rights, virtues, or motives.

Duties are actions demanded by obligations; *moral duties* are actions demanded by moral obligations. Examples of moral duties include parents' obligations to care for their children while young, or nurses' obligations not to harm patients through carelessness or exploitation.

Rights are justified claims; *moral rights* are prima facie claims justified by moral rules, principles, and theories. Commonly held examples of moral rights include the right to health care and the right to life. These rights express morally valid demands made by persons or groups upon others or society. Thus, according to some scholars, wherever there is a right there is also a corresponding obligation, and vice versa. (This thesis is known as the logical correlativity of rights and obligations.) Since rights claims are prima facie, they make strong moral demands, but these demands can be validly overridden by equal or stronger moral demands. For example, the right to life may be justifiably overridden when one person kills another in self-defense.

Virtues are commendable qualities or traits; *moral virtues* are commendable qualities or traits that dispose a person to do what is morally right. With virtues, the focus is on what a person *is* rather than on what a person *does*; that is, the moral worth of a person is judged through that person's character. Rephrased, the emphasis is on "who ought I to be?" rather than on "what ought I to do?" To be morally virtuous, a person's character disposes him or her to exist in accord with moral rules, principles, theories, and ideals. Examples of commonly held virtues include fairness, trustworthiness, patience, generosity, integrity, compassion, and forgiveness. Although moral virtues, when taken alone, are not sufficient for a moral life, they are important for a moral life.

Motives are intentions that underlie actions; *motives involving morality* are intentions that underlie right or wrong purposes. Motives are important because they tell us something about the moral worth of a person. Good motives are morally commendable, whereas evil motives are not. Because good motives may or may not lead to right actions, some persons treat motives and actions as independent of one another. (Utilitarians can also share the preceding views of the importance of virtues and motives.) Having now discussed deontology in general, it is time to focus on particular types of deontology.

Types of Deontology

As with utilitarianism, there are two types of deontology: act and rule. The difference focuses on whether moral demands arising from duty can be applied to specific acts in specific situations or to rules of conduct that determine the rightness or wrongness of an act.

Act Deontology. In act deontology appeals are made directly to conscience, faith, or intuition to determine what is right or obligatory. If rules are used, they serve only as rules of thumb that can be broken if a situation demands it. The act deontologist is concerned with the following question: What effect will my doing *this* act in *this* situation have on my ability to carry out my duty? The emphasis is on action from duty in a particular situation, even if in that particular situation moral rules are violated. In act deontology (as in act utilitarianism) rules can be violated because it is the specific situation that ultimately decides what is right or wrong. It can never be right to act on a rule if one has good reason based on conscience, faith, or intuition that acting on the rule would interfere with the carrying out of one's moral duty in a particular situation.

Act deontology has some strengths. These include sensitivity to particular cases and recognition that abiding by a rule may interfere with one's ability to act from duty, whereas discarding the rule may enhance one's ability to act from duty in a particular situation. Act deontology also has some problems. Perhaps the most troublesome is what would happen to morality if there were no moral guidelines and, instead, persons followed their subjective intuition or conscience. Since intuition and conscience lack external standards, the same or similar acts could result in different moral outcomes. This possibility offends our sense of fair play; that is, equal or comparable moral circumstances should result in equal or comparable, and not different, moral outcomes.

Rule Deontology. In contrast to act deontology, in rule deontology moral rules are important because they constitute binding obligations that transcend individual situations. Rule deontologists turn to moral rules to make appeals about what one ought to do in a particular situation. They then seek to determine how the rules facilitate their ability to act from duty, enabling them to do what is right. Rule deontologists follow moral rules because these rules: (1) serve as standards by which humans perform their moral duties, (2) facilitate systematic resolution of ethical problems, and (3) enhance fairness by applying the same or similar moral standards to similar situations.

The following problem exists, however, with the deontological approach to rules: Which rule(s) should take precedence when two or more absolute rules conflict? Put another way, what rule(s) generate the strongest moral duties? To address this question we turn to the writings of W. D. Ross.

A MIXED ETHICAL THEORY

Underlying Principle: Prima Facie Duties and Actual Duties

W. D. Ross, an English philosopher born in 1877, combined aspects of deontology and utilitarianism. Although Ross is usually categorized as a pluralistic rule deontologist, he did not agree that rules are absolute or that consequences are irrelevant to the moral life. According to Ross, to say that an act is right is not to say that an act is good, in the sense of good maximizing happiness or pleasure. Ross rejected absolute moral rules because it is difficult to know one's duty when two or more of these rules conflict.

To address this problem, Ross developed his principle of prima facie duties and actual duties. Prima facie means at first view or valid at first impression. Therefore, a *prima facie duty* is one that is always binding and right unless it conflicts with equal or stronger duties. When a prima facie duty conflicts with equal or stronger duties, the prima facie duty may be overridden. When the prima facie duty does *not* conflict with equal or stronger duties, it must *without fail* be carried out. For example, one should always tell the truth unless truthfulness comes into conflict with another equal or stronger duty such as the duty not to harm another. If the harm to another would be severe because of truthfulness, then truthfulness may not be a binding moral obligation.

One's moral obligation in the circumstance is called by Ross one's *actual duty* (or duty proper). One's actual duty (i.e., what one morally ought to do) is that duty determined by assessing the various weights of the competing prima facie duties. According to Munson (1983, p. 24), Ross formulated two principles to cope with conflicting duties:

1. When two (and only two) prima facie duties are in conflict, one's duty is that action which is in accord with the stricter prima facie obligation.
2. When several prima facie duties are in conflict, one's duty is

that action which has the greatest balance of prima facie rightness over prima facie wrongness.

This is how Ross explains prima facie duties and actual duties.

W. D. Ross on Prima Facie Duties and Actual Duties[3]

I suggest '*prima facie* duty' or 'conditional duty' as a brief way of
referring to the characteristic (quite distinct from that of being a duty
proper) which an act has, in virtue of being of a certain kind (e.g.,
the keeping of a promise), of being an act which would be a duty
proper if it were not at the same time of another kind which is
morally significant. Whether an act is a duty proper or an actual duty
depends on *all* the morally significant kinds it is an instance of. . . .
(pp. 19–20)

There is nothing arbitrary about these *prima facie* duties.
Each rests on a definite circumstance which cannot seriously be held
to be without moral significance. . . . (p. 20)

The essential defect of the 'ideal utilitarian' theory is that it
ignores, or at least does not do full justice to, the highly personal
character of duty. If the only duty is to produce the maximum of
good, the question who is to have the good—whether it is myself, or
my benefactor, or a person to whom I have made a promise to
confer that good on him, or a mere fellow man to whom I stand in
no special relation—should make no difference to my having a duty
to produce that good. But we are all in fact sure that it makes a vast
difference. . . . (p. 22)

When I ask what it is that makes me in certain cases sure
that I have a *prima facie* duty to do so and so, I find that it lies in the
fact that I have made a promise; when I ask the same question in
another case, I find the answer lies in the fact that I have done a
wrong. And if on reflection I find (as I think I do) that neither of
these reasons is reducible to the other, I must not on any *a priori*
ground assume that such a reduction is possible. . . . (p. 24)

An act is not right because it, being one thing, produces
good results different from itself; it is right because it is itself the
production of a certain state of affairs. Such production is right in
itself, apart from any consequence. (pp. 46–47)

---

[3]**From:** Ross, W. D. (1930). *The right and the good.* Oxford: Oxford University Press.
Reprinted by permission of Oxford University Press, Oxford, England.

Types of Duties

Ross (1930, p. 21) considers the following to be prima facie duties:

Duties of Fidelity. These prima facie duties are concerned with keeping promises and telling the truth.

Duties of Reparation. These prima facie duties are concerned with righting wrongful acts done to others.

Duties of Gratitude. These prima facie duties are concerned with recognizing the services that others have done for us.

Duties of Justice. These prima facie duties are concerned with preventing the unfair distribution of happiness or pleasure to those not meriting them.

Duties of Beneficence. These prima facie duties are concerned with improving the condition of other humans regarding intelligence, virtue, or pleasure.

Duties of Self-Improvement. These prima facie duties are concerned with bettering ourselves regarding intelligence or virtue.

Duties of Nonmaleficence. These prima facie duties are concerned with not harming others.

Regarding the preceding prima facie duties, Ross (1930, pp. 22–23) offers some caveats: (1) The duties are not necessarily complete; (2) they lack the preciseness of language necessary to define all aspects of the duty; and (3) they cannot offer precise guides for distinguishing actual duties from prima facie duties in particular situations. Nevertheless, despite these limitations, Ross's work is important not only because it helps to bridge the gap between utilitarianism and deontology but also because it deals with the common occurrence of a conflict of duties.

Criticisms and Defenses of Deontology

To put deontology into perspective, let us examine how contemporary philosophers have both criticized and defended it. According to Beauchamp (1982, pp. 138–142), criticisms have included: (1) the problem of covert consequential appeals and (2) the problem of nonsystematization.

The Problem of Covert Consequential Appeals. Deontologists vary in the emphasis they place upon consequences, ranging from deontologists who believe that right or wrong actions are determined independent of consequences to those who believe that consequences are relevant to right or wrong acts but are not the sole determiner of them. Particularly in the former situation, however, utilitarians argue that deontologists covertly appeal to consequences in making moral decisions whether or not they recognize or admit it. On this point Mill has criticized Kant, saying that Kant's categorical imperative does in fact deal with the consequences of the universal adoption of a moral action.

Defenders of Kant insist that he is not saying that consequences play no role in deontological moral thinking; rather, what Kant is saying, according to defenders, is that consequences are not the critical determiner of right and wrong actions. This is so because the consequences of an act and the nature of the act often cannot be separated.

The Problem of Nonsystematization. The problem of nonsystematization is leveled toward pluralistic deontological theories. The criticism is that pluralistic deontological theories lack coherence and a unifying principle. As a result deontologists cannot clearly and consistently tell us what makes right acts right. Furthermore, when right acts conflict, deontology does not offer intellectually satisfying reasons for why one right act should take precedence over other right acts. The deontologist's reliance on intuition is troublesome to the utilitarian who finds intuition a weak intellectual basis for moral reasoning.

Defenders of pluralistic deontology say that utilitarians have tried to reduce the moral life to a level of simplicity that does not exist in real life (i.e., the principle of utility). Since morality is complex and untidy, moral philosophers must take these factors into consideration when examining the moral life. Pluralistic deontologists argue that disunity, rather than unity, is inevitable. Furthermore they argue that the principle of prima facie duties is as cohesive a unifying principle for deontology as is the principle of utility for utilitarianism.

In summary, the following can be said about deontology.

- Deontology is a moral theory whose proponents endorse the premise that features of acts other than, or in addition to, their consequences determine the rightness or wrongness of an act.
- Features of acts other than consequences that may determine their rightness or wrongness include duties, rights, virtues, and motives. The right act (i.e., the act that one is morally obligated to follow) is the one that is required by duty. When equally stringent duties conflict, the right act is the one that produces the greatest balance of rightness over wrongness.

- There are two types of deontology. In act deontology appeals are made directly to conscience, faith, or intuition to determine what is right or obligatory in a particular situation. In rule deontology moral rules intervene between an act and one's duty so that one's duty applies to the rule and not to the individual act.
- Problems associated with deontology include its covert appeal to consequences and its unsystematic and intuitive approach to the moral life.

Summary. The focus of this chapter is on helping nurse administrators understand the basics of two classical ethical theories: utilitarianism and deontology. Utilitarianism is a moral theory whose proponents endorse the premise that no acts are right or wrong outside of the consequences produced by the act. The right act is the one whose consequences produce the most net intrinsic value or minimize intrinsic disvalue. In contrast, deontology is a moral theory whose proponents endorse the premise that features of acts other than, or in addition to, their consequences determine the rightness or the wrongness of an act. The right act is the one that is done for the sake of duty. With these two classical ethical theories described, we are ready in Chapter 3 to discuss ethical principles.

REFERENCES

Beauchamp, T. L. (1982). *Philosophical ethics: An introduction to moral philosophy.* New York: McGraw–Hill.

Beauchamp, T. L., & Childress, J. F. (1983). *Principles of biomedical ethics* (2nd ed.). New York: Oxford University Press.

Brody, B. A., & Engelhardt, H. T., Jr. (1987). *Bioethics: Readings & cases.* Englewood Cliffs, NJ: Prentice-Hall.

Ellington, J. W. (1981). Introduction. In I. Kant, *Grounding for the metaphysics of morals* (pp. viii–xvi). Indianapolis: Hackett.

Frankena, W. K. (1973). *Ethics* (2nd ed.). Englewood Cliffs, NJ: Prentice-Hall.

Kant, I. (1981). *Grounding for the metaphysics of morals* (J. W. Ellington, Trans.). Indianapolis: Hackett. (Original work published in German in 1785)

Mathews, J. (1987, February 19). At Beverly Hills eateries, order is: 'Hold the smoke.' *The Washington Post*, p. A3.

Mill, J. S. (1979). *Utilitarianism* (G. Sher, Ed.). Indianapolis: Hackett. (Original work published 1861)

Munson, R. (1983). *Intervention and reflection: Basic issues in medical ethics* (2nd ed.). Belmont, CA: Wadsworth.

Ross, W. D. (1930). *The right and the good.* Oxford: Oxford University Press.

Veatch, R. M., & Fry, S. T. (1987). *Case studies in nursing ethics.* Philadelphia: Lippincott.

3

Ethical Principles: Autonomy, Beneficence, Justice

Mary Cipriano Silva

Knowledge is power.
Francis Bacon

In this chapter nurse administrators are presented with the ethical principles of (1) respect for autonomy, (2) beneficence, and (3) justice. The ethical principle of respect for autonomy focuses on respect for autonomous persons and their actions. The ethical principle of beneficence focuses on noninfliction of harm, prevention of harm, removal of harm, and promotion of good. The ethical principle of justice focuses on giving persons what they are due or owed.

ETHICAL PRINCIPLE OF RESPECT
FOR AUTONOMY

Within the principle of respect for autonomy are the key concepts of (1) respect for persons and (2) autonomy. These two concepts are first defined and then integrated into the ethical principle of respect for autonomy.

The Concept of Respect for Persons

The concept of respect for persons is central to moral philosophy. By respect for persons is meant the capability to recognize, appreciate, and give due weight to other persons' beliefs, capacities, judgments, and perspectives. Engelhardt (1986, p. 86) emphasizes the mutuality of this respect, particularly in secular and pluralistic societies like our own where moral disputes are common. Downie and Telfer (1970, p. 28) speak of an attitude of respect. This attitude encompasses active sympathy (which they consider crucial to the moral life) and a sensitivity to the generalizability of rules (which they define as willingness to consider the applicability of other persons' rules both to themselves and to others). Jameton (1984, p. 125) sees respect for persons as encompassing two principles: (1) People should be treated with empathy (consistent with Downie and Telfer), and (2) people should not be treated as merely means to an end (consistent with Kant). The former principle encompasses an integrated emotional and intellectual awareness of another's position, whereas the latter principle encompasses not exploiting other persons by using them as tools for one's own or others' benefits.

Regarding health care workers and patients, examples of respect for persons include careful listening, genuine concern, individualizing patient care, respecting patient wishes when possible, and addressing patients appropriately. Examples of lack of respect include not listening to patients, feigning concern, treating all patients alike, ignoring patients' reasonable requests, addressing patients by diminutives or in a patronizing tone of voice, or discussing patients in their presence as though they were not there.

Why so much concern with lack of respect and insistence on respect for persons? According to Kant, human beings deserve this respect because of their possession (and their possession alone) of a rational will that allows them to act morally (or as a moral agent). To respect a person, then, is to treat that person as an end and never merely as a means to an end. In Kant's (1785/1981) words:

> Now morality is the condition under which alone a rational being can be an end in himself, for only thereby can be [sic] be a legislating member in the kingdom of ends. Hence morality and humanity, insofar as it is capable of morality, alone have dignity. Skill and diligence in work have a market price; wit, lively imagination, and humor have an affective price; but fidelity to promises and benevolence based on principles (not on instinct) have intrinsic worth. (pp. 40–41) (Reprinted by permission of Hackett Publishing Co., Inc., Indianapolis, Indiana)

According to Beauchamp's (1982a, pp. 129–130) interpretation of Kant, the concept of respect for persons focuses on humans as moral agents. A moral agent not only has the *capacity* to act morally but also *must* act for moral reasons (and not only in accord with the demands of duty). Thus, moral relationships among persons must be characterized by mutual respect. To show respect for persons means to see them as unconditionally worthy human beings, although Kant holds that an immoral judgment need not be respected.

To illustrate, right-to-life advocates often invoke the concept of respect for persons, even when a person is severely mentally or physically handicapped. To them a profoundly mentally retarded person or a comatose person possesses inherent value because each human being, by the nature of that person's humanness, possesses incalculable worth. This incalculable worth is not diminished by disability, no matter how severe. Right-to-life advocates would support life beyond any utilitarian considerations of costs to society. Not all individuals agree with this line of reasoning. Engelhardt (1986, pp. 107–109), for example, would not consider the severely mentally retarded or the comatose to be persons at all because they lack consciousness of self, rationality, and capacity for minimal morality.

In addition to its importance in moral philosophy, the concept of respect for persons is also important in nursing. This concept can be found in the first of eleven principles that constitute the *Code for Nurses with Interpretive Statements* (American Nurses' Association, 1985, p. 2). This principle is as follows: "The nurse provides services with respect for human dignity and the uniqueness of the client, unrestricted by considerations of social or economic status, personal attributes, or the nature of health problems."

The interpretive statement for this principle is reprinted below in its entirety. The language of the statement reflects *both* deontological and utilitarian thinking.

Excerpts from the Code for Nurses[1]

1–1 Respect for Human Dignity. *The fundamental principle of nursing practice is respect for the inherent dignity and worth of every client* [italics added]. Nurses are morally obligated to respect human existence and the individuality of all persons who are the recipients of nursing actions. Nurses therefore must take all reasonable means to protect and preserve human life when there is hope of recovery or reasonable hope of benefit from life-prolonging treatment.

Truth telling and the process of reaching informed choice underlie the exercise of self-determination, which is basic to respect

---

[1]**From:** American Nurses' Association. (1985). *Code for nurses with interpretive statements* (pp. 2–4). Kansas City, MO: Author. Used with permission of the American Nurses' Association.

for persons. Clients should be as fully involved as possible in the planning and implementation of their own health care. Clients have the moral right to determine what will be done with their own person; to be given accurate information, and all the information necessary for making informed judgments; to be assisted with weighing the benefits and burdens of options in their treatment; to accept, refuse, or terminate treatment without coercion; and to be given necessary emotional support. Each nurse has an obligation to be knowledgeable about the moral and legal rights of all clients and to protect and support those rights. In situations in which the client lacks the capacity to make a decision, a surrogate decision maker should be designated.

Individuals are interdependent members of the community. Taking into account both individual rights and the interdependence of persons in decision making, the nurse recognizes those situations in which individual rights to autonomy in health care may temporarily be overridden to preserve the life of the human community; for example, when a disaster demands triage or when an individual presents a direct danger to others. The many variables involved make it imperative that each case be considered with full awareness of the need to preserve the rights and responsibilities of clients and the demands of justice. The suspension of individual rights must always be considered a deviation to be tolerated as briefly as possible.

1–2 Status and Attributes of Clients. The need for health care is universal, transcending all national, ethnic, racial, religious, cultural, political, educational, economic, developmental, personality, role, and sexual differences. Nursing care is delivered without prejudicial behavior. Individual value systems and life-styles should be considered in the planning of health care with and for each client. Attributes of clients influence nursing practice to the extent that they represent factors the nurse must understand, consider, and respect in tailoring care to personal needs and in maintaining the individual's self-respect and dignity.

1–3 The Nature of Health Problems. The nurse's respect for the worth and dignity of the individual human being applies, irrespective of the nature of the health problem. It is reflected in care given the person who is disabled as well as one without disability, the person with long-term illness as well as one with acute illness, the recovering patient as well as one in the last phase of life. This respect extends to all who require the services of the nurse for the promotion of health, the prevention of illness, the restoration of health, the alleviation of suffering, and the provision of supportive care of the dying. The nurse does not act deliberately to terminate the life of any person.

The nurse's concern for human dignity and for the provision of high quality nursing care is not limited by personal attitudes or beliefs. If ethically opposed to interventions in a particular case because of the procedures to be used, the nurse is justified in refusing to participate. Such refusal should be made known in advance and in time for other appropriate arrangements to be made for the client's nursing care. If the nurse becomes involved in such a case and the client's life is in jeopardy, the nurse is obliged to provide for the client's safety, to avoid abandonment, and to withdraw only when assured that alternative sources of nursing care are available to the client.

The measures nurses take to care for the dying client and the client's family emphasize human contact. They enable the client to live with as much physical, emotional, and spiritual comfort as possible, and they maximize the values the client has treasured in life. Nursing care is directed toward the prevention and relief of the suffering commonly associated with the dying process. The nurse may provide interventions to relieve symptoms in the dying client even when the interventions entail substantial risks of hastening death.

1–4 The Setting for Health Care. The nurse adheres to the principle of nondiscriminatory, nonprejudicial care in every situation and endeavors to promote its acceptance by others. The setting shall not determine the nurse's readiness to respect clients and to render or obtain needed services.

In summary, then, respect for persons means the capability to recognize, appreciate, and give due consideration to other persons' beliefs, capacities, judgments, and perspectives. This goal can be accomplished through demonstrating empathy for others and by treating others as ends in themselves and not merely as means to ends. Respect for persons, then, is a concept external to oneself (i.e., how we treat others). As shown in the following section, however, autonomy is a concept integral to the self (i.e., how we govern self).

The Concept of Autonomy

Autonomy can mean either being a self-governing person or acting in a self-governing manner; that is, autonomy can mean self-determining capacities or self-determining actions. According to Faden and Beauchamp (1986, p. 237), "The *capacity* to act autonomously is distinct from *acting* autonomously, and possession of the capacity is no guarantee that an autonomous choice has been or will be made." This distinction between autonomous persons and autonomous actions is necessary because an autonomous person can carry out a nonautonomous action (e.g., a patient with autonomous capacity signs a consent-for-surgery form without reading it). On the other hand, a person generally without the capacity for autonomy can, on occasion, carry out an autonomous action (e.g., when given a choice, a moderately mentally retarded man decides where he wants to live and can justify this decision simply but adequately; however, the man is generally viewed as possessing substantially diminished autonomy to meet the demands of daily living but nonetheless is deserving of respect).

In contrast to the preceding examples, the capacity to act autonomously and acting autonomously can be congruent. One can and often does possess the capacity to act autonomously and then acts autonomously (e.g., a patient with autonomous capacity carefully reads and comprehends a consent-for-surgery form and then signs it freely). (Table 3–1 distinguishes between autonomous persons and autonomous actions.)

TABLE 3–1. CHARACTERISTICS OF AUTONOMOUS PERSONS AND AUTONOMOUS ACTIONS

Autonomous Persons

A person is autonomous only if that person fully or substantially:
1. has the capacity for self-governance,
2. has a coherent and stable set of principles that freely govern his or her actions, and
3. views himself or herself as being capable of carrying out autonomous actions.

Autonomous Actions

According to Faden and Beauchamp (1986, p. 238), a person acts autonomously only if that person fully or substantially acts:
1. with intention,
2. with understanding, and
3. without controlling influences.

Autonomous Persons. Autonomous persons possess the capabilities to plan their lives in accord with a coherent and stable set of principles that they have made their own. In addition, they perceive themselves as being capable of carrying out autonomous actions; that is, they perceive neither internal nor external barriers as preventing them from carrying out their actions. To be an autonomous person, however, these characteristics do not have to be fulfilled completely (as this is an ideal), but they must be fulfilled substantially (Faden & Beauchamp, 1986, pp. 240–241). Substantially autonomous is *conceptually* defined as somewhere between fully autonomous and fully nonautonomous. *In reality*, however, substantially autonomous is defined within the context of specific health care situations. At a minimum, the concept of substantially autonomous must meet the criterion of being realistic enough to be achievable by imperfectly but essentially autonomous persons yet stringent enough to exclude imperfectly but essentially nonautonomous persons.

To illustrate the concept of substantially autonomous, we will examine a research study conducted by Silva (1985) on "Comprehension of Information for Informed Consent by Spouses of Surgical Patients." The study is briefly summarized as follows:

> The adequacy of comprehension of the information needed for informed consent to participate in research on spouse responses to a husband's or wife's general surgery was assessed. Comprehension of information about the research study by 75 spouses was measured by the Informed Consent Questionnaire containing questions on study purpose, time involvement, nature of participation, risks, benefits, voluntariness, confidentiality, and anonymity. The result showed that 72 of the 75 spouses had *adequate comprehension* [italics added] of the information for informed consent. Because adequate comprehension is atypical of most studies, possible reasons for this unexpected result . . . [were] discussed and then explained within a self-determination theory of informed consent. (p. 117)

Although oversimplified, substantially autonomous and adequate comprehension were essentially equated in this study. The Informed Consent Questionnaire (ICQ) contained eight multiple-choice questions focusing on study purpose, time involvement, and so forth, as specified in the preceding paragraph. Possible scores on the ICQ ranged from 0 to 8, with each correct answer receiving a score of 1. A score of 6 or greater was defined as adequate comprehension; a score of 5 or less was defined as inadequate comprehension. The vast majority of the study spouses (96 percent) met the former criterion and were considered as substantially autonomous for the purposes of deciding whether or not to participate in this study.

This example is given to illustrate that the criterion established did not demand perfect comprehension (i.e., all 75 spouses must achieve a perfect score of 8 on the test) but rather a realistic level of comprehension (i.e., all 75 spouses must achieve *at least* a score of 6 on the test). This scoring procedure was an attempt to include into the study only those spouses who were essentially (but not necessarily fully) autonomous for the purposes of a specific informed consent and to exclude those spouses who were essentially (but not necessarily fully) nonautonomous. According to Brock (1987), "Only when . . . misunderstandings or mistakes prove irremediable is there any warrant for a finding of incompetence [in informed consent]" (p. 114). Thus, Brock is not willing to label someone as nonautonomous (incompetent) unless efforts that have been made to increase autonomy fail.

Autonomous Actions. As with autonomous persons, autonomous actions also possess certain characteristics: intentionality, understanding, and voluntariness. (*See* Table 3–1.) These characteristics have been developed in depth by Faden and Beauchamp (1986, pp. 241–262) and are briefly summarized here.

Intentionality. Intentionality is primarily characterized by an action plan. Conceptually this formulation is as follows:

> Whether a given act, X, is intentional, depends on whether in performing X the actor could, upon reflection, say, "I did X as I planned," and in that sense, "I did the 'X' I intended to do." (p. 243)

That is, the person is in charge of the intention and the intention happens as it was planned by the person. To illustrate, suppose a nurse administrator recently fired a staff nurse for using patients' narcotics to support a drug habit. The nurse administrator planned to fire this nurse, and the intended nurse was fired according to the plan. The plan included a personal meeting with the nurse to discuss termination, and the scheduled meeting and termination took place. Therefore, the conditions of intentionality underlying autonomous actions were met.

What if, however, the nurse administrator had planned to reassign the nurse to a position that did not involve drugs, but due to an unfortunate error the nurse was fired? Although in this situation the same outcome occurred (i.e., termination), the nurse administrator could no longer be viewed as engaging in an intentional action because the planned action did not occur as intended.

Another issue surrounding intentionality is whether undesirable or unwanted acts are intentional. Suppose the situation is essentially the same as before: a staff nurse must be fired for using patients' narcotics to support a drug habit. The nurse administrator does not *want* to fire this nurse, however, because the nurse is a friend but does so in accord with the plan. Faden and Beauchamp (1986, pp. 244–246) view the nurse administrator's action as intentional because the act of firing this nurse took precedence over the desire of not wanting to fire a friend. Even though termination was not wanted, it was tolerated.

Understanding. Understanding is important to autonomous actions because an action cannot be autonomous if a person fails to comprehend it. Yet misunderstandings are common problems in health care. One area in which this problem has been documented is informed consent. Silva (1985, p. 118) reviewed research studies on comprehension of information for informed consent and found that "overall, patients who served as research subjects did not adequately comprehend (understand, know, recall) the information presented to them."

To illustrate, Cassileth, Zupkis, Sutton-Smith, and March (1980) asked 200 cancer patients being treated by chemotherapy, radiation, or surgery to recall information they received the previous day related to informed consent. Out of a possible score of 12, the mean test score of the 200 patients was 8.26. Although the vast majority of patients correctly identified their diagnoses, only 60 percent could correctly describe their treatment protocol; only 59 percent could describe the purpose of their treatment; only 55 percent could list one major complication or risk; and only 27 percent could identify one alternative treatment. The authors concluded that many patients were unable to recall major portions of the consent information.

In a similar study conducted by Muss et al. (1979), 100 patients with breast cancer were interviewed 0–24 months after starting chemotherapy to determine their understanding of the purposes, risks, and benefits of treatment as detailed in an informed consent form. Patients averaged 3.44 errors of recall regarding possible side effects. Regarding purposes of chemotherapy, the majority of patients responded incorrectly or were unsure. The authors concluded that this group of patients demonstrated inadequate recall about their disease and therapy.

The results of these two studies are typical of those conducted on comprehension of information for informed consent. Even when one takes into consideration the conceptual and methodological problems inherent in these types of studies, the results ring true; they are congruent with our intuition and experience. Despite our certainty that a problem exists, we remain unclear on whether people understand and on what the term understanding means.

To clarify this concept, Faden and Beauchamp (1986, pp. 248–255) offer the following analysis:

UNDERSTANDING IS A COMPLEX TERM WITH MANY INTERPRETATIONS. These interpretations can be reduced to the following conceptualizations:

1. *Understanding how (to do something)*—suggests possession of a practical competence. "As a nurse administrator, I know how to prepare a budget."
2. *Understanding that (some proposition is true)*—suggests possession of knowledge as a result of believing the knowledge. "I know that this complex of symptoms represents staff nurse burnout."
3. *Understanding what (has been asserted)*—suggests that what has been communicated has been grasped. "I know that you are grieving over the loss of your job."

TO ENGAGE IN AUTONOMOUS ACTIONS, ONE MUST UNDERSTAND THESE ACTIONS. But what is a realistic appraisal of this understanding that is neither too demanding nor too lax? Faden and Beauchamp (1986) offer the following definition:

> A person has a *full* or *complete* understanding of an action if there is a fully *adequate* apprehension of all the *relevant* propositions or statements (those that contribute in any way to obtaining an appreciation of the situation) that correctly describe (1) the nature of the action, and (2) the foreseeable consequences and possible outcomes that might follow as a result of performing and not performing the action. To the extent that this ideal is less than satisfied, an action is based on less than *full* understanding, and thus is less than a fully autonomous action. (p. 252)

This definition has qualifiers (i.e., adequate, relevant) that strike a balance between demanding too much or too little of autonomous actions. It says that full understanding of an action is obtained if there is a fully adequate (*not* perfect) grasp of the relevant (*not* all) aspects of the situation that enable one to make and act upon a decision.

IGNORANCE AND FALSE BELIEFS COMPROMISE AUTONOMOUS ACTIONS. To the extent that an individual's grasp of a proposed action is based on ignorance or false beliefs and, further, to the extent that ignorance and false beliefs hinder understanding of that action, performance of that action is not fully autonomous. To illustrate, suppose the head nurse of an intensive care unit (ICU) and the head nurse of a coronary care unit (CCU) are vying for the same scarce resources (i.e., personnel and supplies). To determine who should receive these resources, the Director of Nursing requests a needs assessment study. After reviewing the results of the study, which the director believes to be true, the bulk of the resources are allocated to the ICU. What the director does not know, however, is that the results of the study had been unfairly slanted in favor of the ICU. Consequently, the director's action is less than fully (or even substantially) autonomous because the decision failed to include this highly relevant knowledge.

ACCURATE INTERPRETATION AND EFFECTIVE COMMUNICATION ARE BASIC TO UNDERSTANDING, AND UNDERSTANDING IS CRUCIAL TO AUTONOMOUS ACTIONS. Accurate interpretation means that a substantially correct correspondence has occurred between what one hears and what was said. According to Faden and Beauchamp (1986):

> If a person claims to understand *that* something, X, is the case, evidence for the truth of X must be shown. But in claiming to understand *what* someone said in asserting the truth of X, one must only show that communication of X has occurred, not that what has been communicated, X, is true. In order to understand in a circumstance of communication, one's formulation or representation of what is said must be substantially *accurate*, but not necessarily *believed*. (p. 255)

To simplify, we can translate the preceding abstract thesis into a concrete example. A nurse administrator says to a colleague, "I understand that classical organization theory is built around several key concepts, including division of labor and span of control." Suppose the colleague responds as follows, "I hear what you are saying. I, too, understand that division of labor and span of control are key concepts in classical organization theory." In this situation, accurate interpretation and effective communication have occurred.

Now suppose that the nurse administrator says the same thing about division of labor and span of control to a beginning staff nurse without administrative knowledge or experience. The staff nurse responds, "*Divisiveness* of labor and span of control are key concepts in classical organization theory." In this situation, an inaccurate interpretation occurred because there was a lack of correspondence between what was said and what was interpreted. This inaccurate interpretation could lead to ineffective communication, which in turn could lead to diminished autonomous actions.

Voluntariness. The third characteristic of autonomous actions is known as a condition of noncontrol; that is, one is not being controlled by others. There is independence of control and no external controls on the action. In contrast, a condition of control means that influences are being exerted. These influences are varied and can include, for example, threats of psychological, physical, or legal harm; monetary incentives; or promises of (or withdrawal of) power, affection, or love. Not all influences on autonomy are controlling, however. Depending on the person or the situation, influences can be trivial or overcome.

The preceding notions are further elaborated upon in the following excerpt.

The Nature of Control and Noncontrol[2]

What, then, do we mean by the terms "controlled act" and "noncontrolled act"? We can begin to address this question by examining the polar extreme of a *completely* or *fully* noncontrolled act. Such acts have either (1) not been the target of an influence attempt, or (2) if they have been the target of an attempt to influence, it was either not successful or it did not deprive the actor in any way of willing what he or she wishes to do or to believe. Thus, a person can be *influenced* without in any way being *controlled* by the influence agent, because the person acts on the basis of what he or she wills rather than on the basis of subjection to the influence agent's will and ends. (pp. 257–258)

By contrast, completely controlled acts are entirely dominated by the will of another; they subject the actor to serve as the means to the other's ends and in no respect to serve the actor's own ends. Person A's action controls an action X of person B if A gets B to do X through irresistible influences that would work even if B, left to his or her own ends, in no way wanted to do X. If a doctor orders a reluctant patient to take a drug, and coerces the patient to compliance, then the patient is under the will of the doctor and is fully controlled. If, by contrast, a physician merely persuades a patient to take a drug that the patient is at first reluctant to take, then the patient wills to take it and is not under the will of the doctor. (p. 258).

There are many in-between cases: For example, suppose the physician has made it clear that he or she will be upset with the patient if the patient does not take the drug, and the patient is intimidated. Although the patient is not convinced that it is the best course to take the medication, which would not be accepted if the

---

[2]**From:** Faden, R. R., & Beauchamp, T. L. (1986). *A history and theory of informed consent.* New York: Oxford University Press.

physician merely offered it as an option, the patient agrees to take the drug because it appears that acceptance will foster a better relationship with the doctor than could otherwise prevail. Here the patient performs the action to a significant extent on the basis of what is willed to personal ends, but only under a heavy *measure* of control by the physician's role, authority, and indeed prescription. Unlike the first case, the patient does not find it overwhelmingly difficult to resist the physician's proposal, but, unlike the second case, it is nonetheless awkward and difficult to resist this rather "controlling" physician. The physician's recommendation is not *ir*resistible, simply *difficult* to resist. (p. 258)

Influences can take three forms: persuasion, manipulation, and coercion. According to Faden and Beauchamp (1986, pp. 258–262), persuasion is never controlling; manipulation may or may not be controlling; and coercion is always controlling.

PERSUASION. This is an intentional and successful influence of an individual through open appeals to reason to accept freely the viewpoint of the persuader. With persuasion, however, choices made and acts performed are noncontrolled.

MANIPULATION. This is an intentional and successful influence of getting an individual to do what the manipulator intended by either (1) noncoercively changing the actual choices available to the individual or (2) nonpersuasively changing the individual's perception of the choices. Manipulation occurs on a continuum between persuasion (never controlling) and coercion (always controlling). Consequently manipulation can occur in degrees and be either substantially noncontrolling, substantially controlling, or somewhere in between.

COERCION. This is an intentional and successful threat of an individual that is so powerful that the individual behaves in a way that he or she finds irresistible. In other words, the individual behaves in a way that he or she would not have behaved if the influence had not been applied. For an influence to be coercive, the person doing the coercing must have (or be perceived as having) the power and ability to carry out the threat. Faden and Beauchamp (1986, p. 339) summarize coercion as follows: "(1) The agent of influence must *intend* to influence the other person by presenting a severe threat; (2) there must be a credible *threat;* and (3) the threat must be *irresistible.*" (For a detailed discussion of coercion, manipulation, and persuasion, see Chapter 10 of Faden and Beauchamp [1986].)

How might these concepts apply to nursing administration? Suppose nurses at a major medical center are threatening to strike because they feel voiceless in matters affecting patient care. Three nurses who work in different critical care areas of the hospital are undecided, however, about whether to strike. They seek consultation with their supervisors, none of whom endorses the strike. Supervisor A gives open and reasoned arguments why Nurse A should not strike. Supervisor A's line of reasoning is that even during a strike the critical care areas of the hospital cannot shut down: nurses have a moral obligation not to abandon severely ill patients without due cause during the time of their hospitalization. Nurse A, as a result of this argument, decides not to strike. This decision is based on the supervisor's persuasion.

Supervisor B in advising Nurse B also argues that nurses have a moral obligation not to abandon severely ill patients. In addition, Supervisor B hints that if Nurse B goes out on strike, Nurse B's relationship with Supervisor B and other supervisors will be strained for some time to come. This latter statement makes Nurse B uncomfortable: it influences the decision not to strike but does not dominate it. Nurse B primarily chooses not to strike to ensure that seriously ill patients received continuous care, but manipulation occurred because Supervisor B indicated that emotional and perhaps other support would be withdrawn if Nurse B went out on strike.

Keeping in mind that manipulation, unlike persuasion and coercion, is on a continuum, one must ask: Was the manipulation substantially controlling, substantially noncontrolling, or somewhere in between? Since the supervisor's comments about strained relationships played an important (but not final determining) role in Nurse B's decision not to strike, the supervisor's influence on Nurse B's capacity for autonomous decision and action was probably somewhere between substantially controlling and substantially noncontrolling. Remember, however, that different nurses might respond differently to Supervisor B's same comments. Some nurses might reject the influence entirely (whereby the manipulation would be substantially noncontrolling) while other nurses might make it the dominant factor in their decision not to strike (whereby the manipulation would be substantially controlling.)

Nurse C approaches Supervisor C, who is very powerful and has the ear of top level nursing and hospital administrators. Supervisor C threatens that Nurse C could be fired for going out on strike, and Nurse C knows that this supervisor could strongly influence that decision. Nurse C is a single parent with two young children. Despite being sympathetic to the cause of the striking nurses, Nurse C does not go out on strike for fear of termination and cannot resist the threat. In this situation, coercion has occurred, and Nurse C's decision not to strike cannot be viewed as an autonomous action.

In summary, then, the concept of autonomy can mean self-determining capacities or self-determining actions. The characteristics of these capacities and actions were highlighted in Table 3–1. The extent to which one or more of these characteristics are lacking affects the degree to which autonomy has been compromised.

The Principle of Respect for Autonomy

In the preceding discussions on respect for persons and on autonomy, we defined two concepts (autonomous persons and autonomous actions) that are associated with, yet different from, the principle of respect for autonomy. This relationship between autonomous persons/actions and respect for autonomy can be stated as follows: Being an autonomous person and acting autonomously are characteristics primarily intrinsic to oneself; however, showing respect for persons and showing respect for autonomous actions are characteristics primarily intrinsic to others (i.e., how one treats an autonomous other person). The principle of respect for autonomy (meant herein to include respect for autonomous persons and/or their actions), focuses on *how* autonomous persons should be treated.

How autonomous persons should be treated has various interpretations (Beauchamp & Childress, 1983, pp. 62–64). For a deontologist of Kantian persuasion, the principle of respect for autonomy has its *primary* emphasis on respect for *persons*. As previously noted, respect for persons stems from the belief that individuals have unconditional worth and should be treated as ends in themselves and not merely as means to an end. Within the Kantian perspective, respect for persons also means respect for their actions; that is, actions of individuals are to be respected because these individuals are the rightful determiners of their destinies. (Although Mill also emphasizes respect for actions, his rationale for this respect is different, as we shall see in the following paragraph.) To summarize, in response to the question of "how do Kantian deontologists treat autonomous persons?," the answer is, "with an attitude of respect."

For a utilitarian of Mill's persuasion, the principle of respect for persons has its *primary* emphasis on respect for autonomous *actions*. In accord with Mill's perspective, insofar as an autonomous individual's actions do not impinge upon the autonomous actions of others, that individual should be free to act without imposed constraints by others.

Simply put, *"Autonomous actions and choices should not be constrained by others"* (Beauchamp & Childress, 1983, p. 62). Mill's qualifier (i.e., insofar as an autonomous individual's actions do not impinge upon the autonomous actions of others) has been omitted in this simpler version because the principle of respect for autonomy, like all moral principles, only has prima facie status and can be overridden by more stringent moral demands. To summarize, in response to the question of "how do utilitarians of Mill's orientation treat autonomous persons?," the answer is, "with noninterference regarding their autonomous actions."

Although the rationale for the principle of respect for autonomy may vary in deontology and in utilitarianism, the outcome in a particular situation may be the same. To illustrate, suppose a male patient admitted to an emergency room for internal bleeding insists that he will not be taken to surgery until he talks with his family doctor, but the doctor is unavailable for two hours. The patient is causing such a ruckus that both a surgical resident and a nursing supervisor are called to assess the situation. After careful examination of the patient, they mutually determine that the patient is rational and that his condition is serious but not critical. Therefore, they agree to honor the patient's request to delay the surgery until the family doctor can be notified; however, their reasons vary. The surgical resident honored the patient's request in the belief that, whenever possible, physicians should not interfere with autonomous patients' requests or actions; the nursing supervisor honored the patient's request in the belief that the patient's dignity would be violated if such a request was denied.

But what if the patient's bleeding is so severe that imminent death would occur without the surgery? This question raises the issue of limits to autonomy or liberty. A treatment of liberty-limiting principles follows.

Liberty-Limiting Principles[3]

Various "moral" principles have been advanced in the attempt to stake out valid grounds for the limitation of individual human liberties. The following four "liberty-limiting principles" have been

[3]**From:** Beauchamp, T. L. (1982b). Ethical theory and bioethics. In T. L. Beauchamp & L. Walters (Eds.), *Contemporary issues in bioethics* (2nd ed., pp. 1–43). Belmont, CA: Wadsworth. © 1982 by Wadsworth, Inc. Reprinted by permission of the publisher.

defended and have played a significant role in recent philosophical controversies:

1. *The Harm Principle*—A person's liberty is justifiably restricted to prevent *harm to others* caused by that person.
2. *The Principle of Paternalism*—A person's liberty is justifiably restricted to prevent *harm to self* caused by that person.
3. *The Principle of Legal Moralism*—A person's liberty is justifiably restricted to prevent that person's *immoral behavior*.
4. *The Offense Principle*—A person's liberty is justifiably restricted to prevent *offense to others* caused by that person. (p. 37)

Each of these four principles represents an attempt to balance liberty and other values. Although different people differently assess the weight of certain values in this balancing process, the harm principle is universally accepted as a valid liberty-limiting principle (despite certain unclarities that surround the notion of a harm). However, much controversy surrounds the other three liberty-limiting principles, and their general validity is widely doubted. (pp. 37–38)

Each of these three "supplementary principles" proclaims that there is a valid limit on individual liberties, and therefore a valid limit on one's *right* to do something. Only one of these supplementary principles is pertinent to many controversies that arise in . . . [health care situations]: paternalism. Here the central problem is whether this form of justification for a restriction of liberty—even if highly qualified—may ever *validly* be invoked—and, if so, how the principle that stands behind this judgment is to be precisely formulated. In order to answer this question, it is necessary to look more closely at the nature of paternalism. (p. 38)

The issue of paternalism (the decision of whether or not to interfere in the affairs of persons who are substantially autonomous) would be raised in the preceding case situation. To recapitulate, a substantially autonomous patient with internal bleeding is refusing surgery until he can talk with his family doctor. Should the surgery be undertaken or not? A conflict such as this leads us to a second ethical principle—the principle of beneficence. It, too, leads to the problem of paternalism.

ETHICAL PRINCIPLE OF BENEFICENCE

According to Frankena (1973), the ethical principle of beneficence includes four components, all of which specify prima facie duties:

1. One ought not to inflict evil or harm (what is bad) [sometimes referred to as nonmaleficence].
2. One ought to prevent evil or harm.
3. One ought to remove evil.
4. One ought to do or promote good. (p. 47)

Frankena (1973, p. 47) however, acknowledges two uncertainties about the principle. First, that disagreement exists about whether or not beneficence is a moral requirement (duty). This disagreement arises because, if beneficence is a moral requirement (duty), then prima facie duty obligates us to prevent harm, remove harm, do good, and not inflict harm. Some persons believe that this demand is too onerous. For example, suppose a campaign is underway to build a Center for Homecare in a community hospital. The purpose of the Center is to facilitate patients' transition from hospital to home. All top level nurse administrators at the hospital have been asked to contribute $500 to help build the Center. Although the nurse administrators can comfortably afford the $500, and although the Center will do good works with the money (i.e., help patients take care of themselves at home), are the nurse administrators morally required to contribute the money? If beneficence is a moral *duty*, then they would be morally required to contribute the money; however, if beneficence is an optional moral *good*, then they would not be morally required to contribute the money, although to do so would be viewed as morally desirable.

Second, Frankena suggests that the components of the principle of beneficence are arranged in a hierarchial order in which, other things being equal, 1 takes precedence over 2, 2 over 3, and 3 over 4. He does not, however, state this position with conviction and not all persons agree with it. Those who disagree with it argue that the weight of the principle is more important than its ordering: For example, prevention of a serious harm should take priority over the infliction of a minor harm. To illustrate, exposing a woman to x-rays during a routine annual mammography may prevent the serious harms that would arise to the woman if breast cancer went undetected.

Not all scholars treat the four components of beneficence in the same way as Frankena. For example, Beauchamp and Childress (1983, pp. 107–108) sometimes treat component 1 (the noninfliction of harm) as a separate ethical principle (the principle of nonmaleficence). They do so because of the distinct moral obligations that nonmaleficence incurs. With this point in mind, we will now examine the concepts of nonmaleficence and beneficence.

The Concept of Nonmaleficence— The Noninfliction of Harm

The notion of "do no harm" is well-entrenched in nursing. It can be found as far back as Florence Nightingale's *Pledge for Nurses* and as recently as the 1985 American Nurses' Association's (ANA) *Code for Nurses with Interpretive Statements*. The Nightingale *Pledge* (cited in Jameton, 1984, p. 316) emphasizes that the nurse will not knowingly administer harmful drugs. The ANA *Code* (1985) stresses that the nurse acts to safeguard clients and protects them from risk of harm.

But what is meant by noninfliction of harm or nonmaleficence? Nonmaleficence (or the duty of nonmaleficence) refers to *not harming* others. Not harming others is a moral action (in contrast to a moral virtue such as nonmalevolence) by which others are spared actual harms. If the duty of nonmaleficence is violated, either through acts of omission or commission, then actual harm such as injuries, damages, impairments, disabilities, or untimely death may occur. For example, if a nurse gives a patient with brittle diabetes the type and amount of insulin the patient is to receive on time and by the route prescribed, the nurse has carried out her duty of nonmaleficence. If the nurse, however, either forgets to give the insulin or gives twice the amount ordered, the nurse has violated her duty of nonmaleficence. Harm would come to the patient in the form of diabetic coma or insulin shock.

In addition to nonmaleficence meaning not harming others, it can also mean not putting others at *risk* for harm. That is, not putting others at risk for harm is a moral action by which others are spared exposure to persons, things, or events that can cause injuries, damages, impairments, disabilities, or untimely death. If the duty of nonmaleficence is violated, then potential or actual harms may occur. Again, if the same nurse caring for another brittle diabetic patient does not remove a nondiabetic dietary tray inadvertently placed on the patient's bedside table, she has placed the patient at risk for harm. By placing the patient at risk for harm, the nurse has violated her duty of nonmaleficence.

One may ask under what conditions nonmaleficence, as a prima facie duty, might be overridden. It might be overridden if proposed goals are important enough to justify the harm or risks to those affected by the goals. Rephrased, using utilitarian thinking, probability and severity of harm or risk of harm are weighed in relation to benefits. Benefits of great worth (e.g., saving the life of a child through risky surgery when no other viable options are available) may also involve (1) harms of high probability and great magnitude (e.g., as a result of the surgery the child would be paralyzed) or (2) great risk of harm (e.g., the child could die during the operation). The point to be made is that one ought not override the duty of nonmaleficence without strong moral justification.

In summary, nonmaleficence has been defined as not harming others and not putting others at risk of harm. The prima facie duty of nonmaleficence may always be overridden if benefits are powerful enough to justify the harm or risk.

The Concept of Beneficence—The Prevention of Harm, the Removal of Harm, and the Promotion of Good

In addition to not inflicting harm or placing others at risk for harm, other important concepts in nursing are the prevention of harm, the removal of harm, and the promotion of good. Examples of these beneficent concepts can be found in excerpts from the International Council of Nurses' (1973) *Code for Nurses: Ethical Concepts Applied to Nursing:*

- The fundamental responsibility of the nurse is fourfold: to promote health, to prevent illness, to restore health and to alleviate suffering. (p. 1)
- The nurse shares with other citizens the responsibility for initiating and supporting action to meet the health and social needs of the public. (p. 2)

These excerpts highlight nurses' other-regarding focus, that is, their focus on helping others achieve and maintain health. A beneficent goal such as this can be better understood through analysis of two principles inherent in beneficence: (1) the principle of positive beneficence and (2) the principle of balancing benefits and harms (Beauchamp & Childress, 1983, pp. 149–179).

The Principle of Positive Beneficence. The concept that human beings should positively benefit other human beings (the principle of positive beneficence) is well-established in the health care professions. Positively benefiting includes the three components of *prevention of harm, removal of harm,* and *promotion of good.* By prevention of harm is meant the taking of advanced measures against some possible or probable event (e.g., nurses frequently turn comatose patients to prevent decubitus ulcers). By removal of harm is meant the elimination of an existing situation where injury, damage, impairment, or disability has occurred (e.g., an administrator fires a nurse who has injured patients through incompetence). By promotion of good is meant the contribution to the welfare of others (e.g., an administrator establishes a health hot line for the elderly).

Whether beneficence is a moral duty is admittedly controversial because of the strong moral obligations that duties incur. The notion of beneficence as duty incurs these strong moral obligations because it makes positive benefiting a moral requirement. This is quite different from saying that beneficence is a moral virtue or a moral ideal—neither of which places the demands on beneficence that duties do. That is, if beneficence is a duty, it always obligates us to prevent harm, remove harm, or do good. These requirements are troublesome to some scholars for they seem too demanding. Consequently these scholars prefer to see beneficence conceptualized as a virtuous or ideal act rather than as a duty.

To find some middle ground in this controversy, Beauchamp and Childress (1983), building on D'Arcy's (1963) work, have conceptualized the duty of beneficence as follows:

> X has a duty of beneficence toward Y *only* [italics added] if each of the following conditions is satisfied:
>
> 1. Y is at risk of significant loss or damage,
> 2. X's action is needed to prevent this loss,
> 3. X's action would probably prevent it,
> 4. X's action would not present significant risk to X, and
> 5. the benefit that Y will probably gain outweighs any harms that X is likely to suffer. (p. 153)

Let us illustrate this abstract conceptualization with a concrete example, where X represents A, the Director of Nursing of a 250-bed community hospital, and Y represents B, a head nurse. B comes to Director A's office upset because a physician has threatened loss of B's job because B supported an autonomous patient's right to make a decision to refuse a medical intervention. (*Y is at risk of significant loss or damage.*) Within this facility, the hiring and firing of nursing personnel ultimately is the responsibility of the Director of Nursing. (*X's action is needed to prevent this loss and would probably prevent it.*) Director A knows from past experience that although A will lose popularity with this physician (or some others) for supporting the head nurse, A is not in jeopardy of losing the directorship. (*X's action would not present signifi-cant risk to X.*) The benefit to B (job security) is greater than the harm (unpopularity with some physicians) that A will experience. (*The benefit that Y will probably gain outweighs any harms that X is likely to suffer.*)

In the preceding situation, then, the Director of Nursing has a duty to protect the head nurse's job. If all of the preceding criteria were not met, however, the Director of Nursing technically would not have a moral duty to protect the head nurse's job, but it would be morally virtuous to do so. At a minimum, the Director of Nursing must take a course of action that is morally justifiable. (*See* Chapter 1 for a review of moral justification.)

In summary, scholars disagree on whether the principle of positive beneficence is a duty, however, there is little disagreement that actions based on beneficence are morally good. Failure to benefit others when one is in a position to do so violates well-established moral traditions in philosophy, nursing, medicine, and public health. Thus, regarding be-neficence, it is important to distinguish between a general moral duty and a moral duty intrinsic to one's role obligations. A general moral duty of beneficence may be less stringent than a role-obligated moral duty of beneficence.

The Principle of Balancing Benefits and Harms. The moral life would be simpler if one could produce benefits *and* avoid harms. Since benefits often occur with harms, a balancing principle is needed. Such a principle can be formulated as follows: "We . . . have a moral duty to weigh and balance possible benefits against possible harms in order to maximize benefits and minimize risks of harm" (Beauchamp & Childress, 1983, p. 159). The requirements for beneficence do not in and of themselves con-stitute a morally justifiable course of action if serious risks are unavoid-able in the attempt to produce benefits. As with the principle of positive beneficence, the principle of balancing benefits and harms has prima fa-cie status. That is, if balancing benefits and harms is not overridden by other principles, it is morally permissible to perform an action if the risks of the procedure are reasonable (and personally and/or socially accept-able) when compared with the anticipated benefits.

Although the principle sounds straightforward, it is difficult to implement. For example, what constitutes reasonable risks? What con-stitutes benefits? When do benefits outweigh risks? How should bene-fits and costs be distributed? Who should pay for benefits or harms incurred as a result of risks? Who should govern decisions involving benefits and risks?

The Problem of Paternalism

Who should govern decisions brings us to the problem of paternalism. In the general vernacular paternalism means that, in the governance of their decisions, authority figures treat those under their control in a fatherly (parental) manner. In ethical theory paternalism means that one's wishes or intended actions are overridden for beneficent reasons without a person's consent. The paternalistic approach implies: (1) intention to be helpful and (2) intervention to override the decisions of others in order to help them or to prevent harm to them. Whether these interventions are morally justified is the problem of paternalism. Paternalism focuses on the claim that beneficence may override autonomy.

Paternalism is common both in society and in health care, as illustrated in the following.

Paternalism in Society and in Health Care[4]

Several writers have argued that paternalism is pervasively present in modern society; many actions, rules, and laws are commonly justified by appeal to a paternalistic principle. Examples in medicine include court orders for blood transfusions when patients have refused them, involuntary commitment to institutions for treatment, intervention to stop "rational" suicides, resuscitating patients who have asked not to be resuscitated, withholding medical information that patients have requested, denial of an innovative therapy to someone who wishes to try it, and some government efforts to promote health. Other health-related examples include laws requiring motorcyclists to wear helmets and motorists to wear seat belts and the regulations of governmental agencies such as the Food and Drug Administration that prevent people from purchasing possibly harmful or inefficacious drugs and chemicals. In all cases the motivation is the beneficent promotion of health and welfare.

In the case of *medical* paternalism, it is often said that the patient–physician relationship is essentially paternalistic. This view is held because patients can be so ill that their judgments or voluntary abilities are significantly affected, or because they may be incapable

---

[4]**From:** Beauchamp, T. L. (1982b). Ethical theory and bioethics. In T. L. Beauchamp & L. Walters (Eds.), *Contemporary issues in bioethics* (2nd ed., pp. 1–43). Belmont, CA: Wadsworth. © 1982 by Wadsworth, Inc. Reprinted by permission of the publisher.

of grasping important information about their case, thus leaving them in no position to reach carefully reasoned decisions about their medical treatment. Illness, injury, depression, fear, the threat of death, and traditional staples of the medical profession such as drugs may overwhelm patients, so that their ability to ascertain their own best interests is in doubt. Moreover, every increase in illness, ignorance, and quantity of medication can increase the patient's dependence on his or her physician. Also, physicians commonly encourage patients with "innocent lies" intended to raise their spirits—when, in fact, matters are either hopeless or beyond the physician's capacities. Hospitals and the medical profession thus seem immersed in a paternalistic orientation.

The paternalism of the medical profession has been under attack in recent years, especially by defenders of patient autonomy. They hold that physicians intervene too often and assume too much control over their patients' choices. Many recent philosophical, legal, and medical writings have reflected this harsh judgment of the profession. Philosophers and lawyers have tended to support the view that patient autonomy is the decisive factor in the patient–physician relationship and that interventions can be valid only when patients are in some measure unable to make voluntary choices or to perform voluntary actions. Physicians too have increasingly criticized authoritarianism in their profession. In fact, a recent draft of principles of ethics of the American Medical Association asserted that "paternalism by the profession is no longer appropriate." (pp. 38–39)

Although the emphasis in the preceding excerpt is on the medical profession, many of the comments also hold for the nursing profession. In general, nurses are reluctant to allow autonomous patients to make health care decisions that may harm or not benefit them. Yet the preamble to the American Nurses' Association's (1985, p. i) *Code for Nurses with Interpretive Statements* stresses that "clients themselves are the primary decision makers in matters concerning their own health, treatment, and well-being" and that the nurse's role is to support clients' self-determination. The *Code*, however, does not elucidate under what conditions restraints on self-determination may be morally justifiable. To clarify this point, two types of paternalism are discussed: (1) Strong paternalism is the justifiable limitation of the liberty of persons whose choices are voluntary and informed; (2) weak paternalism is the justifiable limitation of the liberty of persons whose choices are substantially or questionably nonvoluntary and/or uninformed.

With paternalism, a person's liberty is justifiably limited to prevent that person from harming self. If a person's liberty is justifiably limited to prevent harm to others, the harm principle rather than paternalism is invoked.

Strong Paternalism. Under what circumstances might strong paternalism be justified? Some persons believe strong paternalism is justified in cases where autonomous persons plan to embark on courses of actions that are profoundly dangerous or harmful to themselves. Others believe strong paternalism is justified in situations where autonomous persons are (or feel) powerless, where a substantial knowledge gap exists between clients and persons providing services to clients, or where persons refuse to make a decision and insist that others make it. Most persons believe, however, that when strong paternalism is invoked, it requires a heavy burden of moral justification.

To illustrate, let us examine a commonplace example in nursing: the use of side rails for preoperatively sedated patients. After receiving his preoperative medicine, C, a 23-year-old male athlete scheduled for a hernia repair, states that he does not want the side rails up. C is of clear mind and understands why the rule is required; however, C does not feel the rule should apply to him because he is not the least bit drowsy from the preoperative medication, and he has no intention of falling out of bed. After considerable discussion between the nurse and patient, the nurse responsible for C's care puts the side rails up. The justification is as follows: C is not drowsy because he has just received the preoperative medication, and its effects have not occurred. Furthermore, if he follows the typical pattern of patients receiving this medication in this dosage, he will become drowsy very quickly. A drowsy patient is at risk for a fall. Since there is no family at the hospital to remain with the patient, and since the nurses on the unit are exceptionally busy, no one can constantly stay with C to monitor his level of alertness. Under these circumstances the patient must be protected from the potential harm of a fall despite the fact that he does not want this protection. It is important to emphasize that the nurse restricted this autonomous patient's liberty based on a morally justified reason (i.e., protection of the patient from potential harm) and *not* as a hedge against liability or for protection from criticism.

The preceding example illustrates strong paternalism because the free choice of an alert and informed patient was overridden by the nurse, thus limiting the patient's liberty in an effort to prevent harm to him. Thereby the principle of beneficence overrode the principle of autonomy. Whereas some professionals would be in agreement with the nurse's action, others might argue that the circumstances were not serious enough to warrant impingement on an alert and informed patient's autonomy. Strong paternalism needs strong moral justification.

Weak Paternalism. Although easier to justify morally than strong paternalism, weak paternalism also must meet stringent criteria. According to Beauchamp and Childress (1983), paternalism can only be justified if:

1. The harms prevented from occurring or the benefit provided to the person outweighs the loss of independence or the sense of invasion suffered by the interference,
2. The person's condition seriously limits his or her ability to choose autonomously, and
3. It is universally justified under relevantly similar circumstances always to treat persons in this way. (p. 172)

The second criterion is the one most frequently invoked in situations of weak paternalism. If severe enough, conditions frequently considered capable of limiting autonomous choice include mental retardation, depression, drug addiction, and the effects of strokes.

To illustrate, let us examine another commonplace example in nursing: the patient whose mental faculties have been moderately or severely impaired. Suppose D, a patient with a stroke, wants to leave the hospital against medical advice because "the hospital isn't helping him." The nurse's assessment of D shows moderate loss of motion on his dominant side, slurred speech, impaired judgment, and labile emotions. The loss of motion and slurred speech raise questions about D's ability to communicate his needs clearly. The impaired judgment and emotional lability raise questions about D's ability to make a rational decision about his discharge. If D left the hospital against medical advice, the nurse is convinced that harm would come to him. He is unable to care for himself without supervision, and he has no family to care for him. Consequently, the nurse does not support his request to leave the hospital against medical advice.

Is the nurse's paternalistic action morally justified? Let us examine this question in terms of the three preceding Beauchamp and Childress criteria:

The Harms Prevented Outweigh the Sense of Invasion. Restricting D's freedom to return to his home is a serious invasion of his liberty, but potential harms to him by not restricting his freedom are also serious. Since D cannot care for himself independently, he would be unable to meet many of his basic needs, including adequate nutrition. Inability to meet nutritional needs over time could result in malnourishment or even death. Therefore potential harms seem to outweigh the sense of invasion.

The Person's Condition Limits Autonomous Choice. D's significantly impaired thought processes and emotional lability limit his autonomous choices.

The Circumstances Are Generalizable. It would seem morally justifiable (based on the preceding) to treat not only D but all persons in circumstances like D's in the same way (i.e., override their decision to return home against medical advice in order to prevent them from causing harm to themselves). Consequently we conclude that the nurse's weak paternalism can be morally justified. Because it can be morally justified, however, does not necessarily mean that all nurses agree with it. Morally justifiable arguments against weak paternalism and for autonomy can also be mounted by strong autonomy advocates.

In summary, the principle of beneficence is concerned with the noninfliction of harm (nonmaleficence) and positive beneficence (the prevention of harm, the removal of harm, and the promotion of good). It is also concerned with balancing benefits against harms in order to maximize benefits and minimize risk of harm. Sometimes when maximizing benefits and minimizing risk of harm, there are also questions of justice.

ETHICAL PRINCIPLE OF JUSTICE

Simply stated, justice means giving others their due (Jameton, 1984, p. 130). This meaning is rooted in the ancient concept of *desert,* or giving others what they deserve or can legitimately claim. What persons deserve may be punishments, rewards, or burdens. Nurse administrators who defraud their institutions deserve punishment. Nurse administrators who promote quality care deserve rewards. Nurse administrators who are U.S. citizens accept the burden of taxation.

Matters of justice are not always easy; in fact, they can cause considerable controversy. An example of a contemporary controversy surrounding justice is the recent Supreme Court decision to uphold affirmative action hiring (Kamen, 1987, March 26). On March 25, 1987 the Supreme Court ruled 6 to 3 that employers may promote minorities and women ahead of white males, even when no evidence of prior discrimination by the employer existed. The employer must be able to point to an apparent imbalance, however, in the presence of minorities and women in jobs that are traditionally segregated.

This Supreme Court decision grew out of a 1981 job dispute where a Ms Joyce was promoted to a road dispatcher job ahead of a Mr Johnson, although Johnson scored two points higher on an oral examination. The following chain of events occurred:

1. Johnson sued, saying he was illegally denied promotion because of reverse discrimination based on gender.
2. The county said Joyce was properly promoted in accord with an affirmative action plan to correct an imbalance in the county's work force. (According to the county, in 1981 there were no women in any of the 238 positions in the road dispatcher job category.)
3. A district court ruled in Johnson's favor saying gender could not be taken into account, *unless* the county had been shown to have engaged in past discrimination against women.
4. The preceding decision was reversed by the 9th U.S. Circuit Court of Appeals, and Johnson appealed.
5. The Supreme Court ruled in favor of Joyce, saying that Johnson had no absolute claim on the road dispatcher position, as seven of the candidates were qualified and eligible. Thus the agency director had the authority to promote any one of them.

In this situation, both Ms Joyce and Mr Johnson made justice-based claims to the road dispatcher job, with Ms Joyce viewing "justice as desert" and Mr Johnson viewing "justice as equality of treatment." Ms Joyce and the Supreme Court justices who upheld the affirmative action hiring felt justice was served; that is, existing gender imbalances in a system can now be corrected. Mr Johnson and the Supreme Court justices who did not support the ruling felt justice was ill served; that is, the ruling guarantees that gender may now be used as a basis for determination of employment, violating the equality inherent in non-discrimination. Although it is too early to predict the long-term consequences of the Supreme Court decision, the rendering of justice in cases just as this one is not easy.

The Formal Principle of Justice

Although justice can be perceived differently, there is one common basic principle. Attributed to Aristotle, the *formal principle of justice* asserts that "equals ought to be treated equally and unequals unequally" (Beauchamp, 1982a, p. 223). Put another way, it means that persons equal in characteristic X should be treated equally, whereas persons unequal in characteristic X should be treated unequally. For example, if two (or more) staff nurses on a given unit have a drug dependency problem so severe as to interfere with safe patient care, they should receive equal or comparable penalties (and/or treatments) for the problem. If the other staff nurses do not have a drug dependency problem, then they should not receive the penalties (and/or the treatments) of the drug-dependent nurses. Frankena (1973, p. 49) puts it well: "The paradigm case of injustice is that in which there are two similar individuals in similar circumstances and one of them is treated better or worse than the other."

Although the formal principle of justice is useful, it is also limiting because it does not specify: (1) Who is equal and who is unequal, and (2) what are morally relevant differences among persons that allow one to determine what each person is due.

Material Principles of Justice

To overcome these problems, theories of justice incorporate material principles of justice. These identify relevant moral characteristics that serve as a basis for determining what a person is owed or due. Material principles of justice are typically applied to *distributive justice*, which deals with competing claims for scarce resources. Therefore, distributive justice is concerned with the equitable distribution of a society's benefits and burdens. An example of a societal benefit is accessible health care; an example of a societal burden is taxes.

In highlighting the relationship between distributive justice and nursing, Silva (1984) argues that:

> [Nurses] . . . have a moral responsibility to identify and resolve ethical issues related to distributive justice because (a) issues of distributive justice affect the type and amount of total societal resources available for health care; (b) the method by which this health care (including nursing care) is allocated affects the public good; and (c) benefiting and not harming the public good in matters of health are moral obligations inherent in the social contract between nursing and society. (p. 12)

This social contract stipulates that society grants a profession autonomy and authority over its practice in return for that profession's safeguarding of the public trust (American Nurses' Association, 1980,

p. 7). Part of this trust includes the responsibility of nurse administrators to distribute equitably nursing's benefits and burdens. To do so, material principles of justice must be considered.

Examples of material principles of justice identified by Jameton (1984, p. 133) and considered morally relevant to distributive justice include the following:

1. To each person equally. (e.g., All beginning staff nurses should receive the same salary.)
2. To each person according to merit. (e.g., Staff nurses whose performances are outstanding should receive more salary than staff nurses whose performances are mediocre.)
3. To each person according to past or future societal contributions. (e.g., Staff nurses who have made a substantial past contribution to improved patient care should have this contribution reflected in their salaries.)
4. To each person according to what can be acquired in a free market. (e.g., Staff nurses who work in high cost-of-living areas should receive more salary than staff nurses who work in low cost-of-living areas.)
5. To each person according to need. (e.g., Staff nurses who are in legitimate financial distress should have this distress considered in their salaries.)
6. To each person according to. . . (State other morally relevant characteristics.)

Notice that the relevant characteristics on which scarce resources are distributed must be *morally* relevant ones, such as the six preceding ones. Morally relevant characteristics are those that bear on the goodness or badness of an individual's life (Frankena, 1973, p. 51). Differences among persons such as height, weight, or degree of attractiveness, for example, do not constitute morally relevant differences on which to base the allocation of scarce societal resources. On the other hand, what does constitute morally relevant differences, and which morally relevant differences take precedence when material principles of justice are in conflict, are not easy questions to answer.

Although nurse administrators have a basic moral obligation to equitably distribute scarce nursing resources, this obligation is not always binding if the obligation conflicts with equal or stronger ones: The principle of distributive justice is a prima facie one that can be overruled by other moral principles such as autonomy or beneficence.

Conflicts Among Ethical Principles[5]

The principles of autonomy and beneficence that lie at the
foundations of justice will spawn conflicts within any portrayal of a
just allocation of health care resources. . . .
    These fundamental conflicts between respecting the freedom
and achieving the best interests of persons are made worse by
commitments to goals that, if pursued without qualification, lead to
even more elaborate tensions within any concrete vision of a just
health care system. Consider the following four goals that are at
loggerheads.

1. The provision of the best possible care for all
2. The provision of equal care for all
3. Freedom of choice on the part of health care provider and
   consumer
4. Containment of health care costs

One cannot provide the best possible health for all and contain the
cost of health care. One cannot provide equal health care for all and
maintain freedom in the choice of health care provider and
consumer. For that matter, one cannot maintain freedom in the
choice of health care services while containing the costs of health
care. One also may not be able to provide all with equal health care
that is at the same time the very best care because of limits on the
resources themselves. These tensions spring not only from a conflict
between freedom and beneficence, but from competing views of
what it means to pursue and achieve the good in health care (e.g., is
it more important to provide equal care to all or the best possible
care to the least well-off class?). (pp. 336–337)

    To illustrate, let us examine the conflict between the provision of
the best possible care for all and containment of health care costs. G is a
registered nurse typically responsible for the care of six surgical patients. G's goal is to give these patients the best possible care. For

---

[5]**From:** Engelhardt, H. T., Jr. (1986). *The foundations of bioethics*. New York: Oxford
University Press.

reasons of cost-containment, however, H, the Director of Nursing in G's agency has just received a mandate to cut the budget by 10 percent. This means H can no longer afford to hire temporary or new nursing personnel. One of the recommendations that Director H makes is that whenever possible staff nurses are to increase the number of patients they care for by one. This recommendation upsets G for fear of compromising the quality of care given to patients. G would have less time to prevent complications of surgery or to give patients extra attention. G is also concerned that harm could come to patients because they cannot be monitored closely postoperatively. In short, Nurse G's concerns focus on the principle of beneficence. On the other hand, the Director H's concerns focus on the principle of justice: how equitably to distribute the burden of too many patients with too few nurses. In situations such as these a balance must be attained between beneficence and justice. Quality of care may have to be sacrificed but not to the degree where harm comes to patients. A mechanism for accomplishing this goal is an equitable redistribution of the nurse–patient ratio.

In further clarifying material principles of justice, one should note that some, but not all, are mutually exclusive. The material principles of justice that specify "to each person according to merit" and "to each person according to societal contribution" are more compatible with one another than they are with the material principle of justice that specifies "to each person equally." Material principles of justice that are not mutually exclusive may be used in combination when trying to determine what persons are owed or due. For example, all staff nurses at a given hospital could receive the same cost-of-living salary increase (to each person equally), but some of these staff nurses who meet high performance standards could also receive additional salary (to each person according to merit).

Perspectives on Distributive Justice

How material principles of justice and ethical principles interrelate can be viewed within four theoretical perspectives on distributive justice: libertarian, utilitarian, egalitarian, and need-based perspectives. Each of these theoretical perspectives gives priority to certain ethical principles over others. These four perspectives represent one approach to organizing theories of distributive justice.[6]

---

[6]Discussion of the four theoretical perspectives are from "Ethics, Scarce Resources, and the Nurse Executive" by M. C. Silva, 1984, *Nursing Economic$*, 2, 13–16. Copyright 1984 by Anthony J. Jannetti, Inc., publisher *Nursing Economic$*. Modified with permission.

The Libertarian Perspective on Distributive Justice. According to Beauchamp (1982a, pp. 230–232), libertarians focus primarily on the problems of the just allocation of economic benefits and burdens. There is a strong advocacy for mechanisms that ensure that rights are recognized in economic practice, in particular, rights to social and economic liberty. Mechanisms to attain these rights are characteristically those that govern gains and acquisitions in free market or capitalist systems. These free market or capitalist systems are characterized by individuals who freely enter and freely withdraw from economic arrangements in accord with their own interests, but with the intent that their self-interests collectively benefit the larger society. The key herein is that these individuals have a substantial degree of economic freedom. Libertarians believe that persons who freely produce more should receive more economic benefits than persons who produce less, even if this process leads to inequalities of wealth in a society.

In the libertarian perspective, free choice is a central concept. Thus, libertarians place a high value on autonomy and the ethical principle of autonomy. They believe that people freely choose to contribute as they wish to economic matters, and that this freedom should not be interfered with in autonomous persons. To interfere with this freedom would demonstrate lack of respect for persons. In fact, libertarians would go so far as to say that a serious violation of justice would occur if individuals a priori were deemed deserving of equal economic returns.

Based on this discussion, a number of material principles of justice seem appropriate to the libertarian perspective. Examples include:

- To each person according to that person's rights.
- To each person according to individual effort.
- To each person according to societal contribution.

Strengths of the libertarian perspective are its commitment to liberty and a strong respect for persons and for individual differences among them. Opponents of the libertarian perspective argue that the allocation of societal benefits and burdens strictly and only according to rights, effort, or societal contribution would be unjust because it is unfair. It is unfair because many of the characteristics that comprise individual differences are not of the individual's doing but rather a matter of genetics or luck. Therefore, according to opponents, the least advantaged members of society would suffer unduly under libertarianism. A just (fair) society would not tolerate this inequity. Furthermore, the libertarian perspective could foster a society where, on the whole, some few individuals would benefit greatly from many economic benefits and few economic burdens, whereas the rest of society would receive few benefits and many burdens.

The Utilitarian Perspective on Distributive Justice. According to Beauchamp (1982a, pp. 80–84), the utilitarian perspective can be reduced to two major theses: (1) An action is right if it leads to the greatest possible balance of good consequences or to the least possible balance of bad consequences for all persons involved with the action; and (2) that which maximizes the good (i.e., ensures the best consequences) determines what is right to do.

Therefore to utilitarians, no act is right or wrong in itself outside of the consequences. That is, the intrinsic value of each consequence for all persons involved becomes the morally relevant factor that determines an act's right-making or wrong-making characteristics. In addition, according to Mill (1861/1979, p. 16), when a decision must be made between one's own happiness and that of others, utilitarianism requires a person to invoke the golden rule. When these perspectives on utilitarianism are applied to distributive justice, the formulation is often stated as follows: (1) Identify methods to allocate a societal resource; (2) determine the benefit and cost consequences of each method based on its intrinsic value; and (3) choose the course of action that maximizes the net benefit over cost for all involved.

The utilitarian perspective holds the doing of good and the prevention of harm as its central concepts. Thus utilitarians place a high value on the ethical principle of beneficence. This is because the consequence of any act (and thus its rightness) is evaluated in terms of its good or its ability to prevent harm.

Material principles of justice appropriate to the utilitarian perspective include:

- To do unto each person as you would be done to.
- To each person according to the greatest good for the greatest number.

Strengths of the utilitarian perspective include a strong sense of community, a concern for doing as much good as possible for the largest number of people, and a practical approach to determining the rightness and wrongness of an act through assessing consequences.

Problems with the utilitarian perspective include the possibility that the interests of the majority could override the interests of the minority, that individual needs could become subservient to group needs, that good and the prevention of harm cannot be easily quantified, and that utilitarianism does not tell us how the aggregate good derived from its formulations should be distributed.

The Egalitarian Perspective on Distributive Justice. Equality plays a central role in egalitarian theories of justice, thus, egalitarians place a high value on the ethical principle of justice as equality. According to Veatch (1981, p. 265), who holds a controversial viewpoint, justice requires the "equality of net welfare for individuals." What this means is that over the course of a lifetime there should be a balanced distribution of hardships and benefits (Beauchamp & Pinkard, 1983, p. 133). Some persons may have about an average amount of both hardships and benefits, whereas others may experience outstanding benefits but also severe hardships. Egalitarianism does not demand uniformity, but it does demand comparability over time. It differs from the libertarian and the utilitarian perspectives because it takes into account equally the individuality of each member of society (Veatch, 1981, p. 266).

A less controversial egalitarian perspective on justice is held by John Rawls. Rawls (1971) formalized his thoughts on justice in the following two principles.

"**First:** each person is to have an equal right to the most extensive basic liberty compatible with a similar liberty for others. **Second:** social and economic inequities are to be arranged so that they are both (a) reasonably expected to be to everyone's advantage, and (b) attached to positions and offices open to all." (p. 60)

Rawls states and defends his two principles of justice in the following excerpt.

Principles of Justice[7]

By way of general comment, these principles primarily apply, as I have said, to the basic structure of society. They are to govern the assignment of rights and duties and to regulate the distribution of social and economic advantages. As their formulation suggests, these principles presuppose that the social structure can be divided into two more or less distinct parts, the first principle applying to the one, the second to the other. They distinguish between those aspects of the social system that define and secure the equal liberties of citizenship and those that specify and establish social and economic inequalities. The basic liberties of citizens are, roughly speaking, political liberty (the right to vote and to be eligible for public office) together with freedom of speech and assembly; liberty of conscience and freedom of thought; freedom of the person along with the right to hold (personal) property; and freedom from arbitrary arrest and seizure as defined by the concept of the rule of law. These liberties are all required to be equal by the first principle, since citizens of a just society are to have the same basic rights.

The second principle applies, in the first approximation, to the distribution of income and wealth and to the design of organizations that make use of differences in authority and responsibility, or chains of command. *While the distribution of wealth and income need not be equal, it must be to everyone's advantage* [italics added], and at the same time, positions of authority and offices of command must be accessible to all. One applies the second principle by holding positions open, and then, subject to this constraint, arranges social and economic inequalities so that everyone benefits.

These principles are to be arranged in a serial order with the first principle prior to the second. This ordering means that a departure from the institutions of equal liberty required by the first principle cannot be justified by, or compensated for, by greater social and economic advantages. The distribution of wealth and income, and the hierarchies of authority, must be consistent with both the liberties of equal citizenship and equality of opportunity. (p. 61)

It is clear that these principles are rather specific in their content, and their acceptance rests on certain assumptions that I must eventually try to explain and justify. A theory of justice depends upon a theory of society in ways that will become evident as we proceed. For the present, it should be observed that the two principles (and this holds for all formulations) are a special case of a more general conception of justice that can be expressed as follows.

> All social values—liberty and opportunity, income and wealth, and the bases of self-respect—are to be distributed equally unless an unequal distribution of any, or all, of these values is to everyone's advantage.

Injustice, then, is simply inequalities that are not to the benefit of all. (p. 62)

An important notion in Rawls's writing is that economic and social inequalities are to be ordered so that they are reasonably expected to be to everyone's advantage, including the least advantaged members of society. This suggests that the distribution of wealth in a society does not have to be perfectly equal if everyone benefits. For example, if certain advantaged groups in a society were given substantial economic incentives to contribute to programs that materially assisted those in need of jobs to obtain jobs, then justice would be served if both groups benefited.

Material principles of justice appropriate to the egalitarian perspective include:

- To each person an equal share.
- To each person a comparable share.

Strengths of the egalitarian perspective include its ability to take into account the needs of all members of society equally when allocating benefits and burdens, its commitment to democratic principles, and its sensitivity to the undesirable psychological effects generated when substantial inequalities occur in a society's net benefits or burdens.

Opponents of the egalitarian perspective argue that attainment of equality of net welfare is impossible, that the egalitarian position is one whose basic grounding is in envy of others, that the egalitarian perspective would diminish human incentives, and that the egalitarian perspective forcibly extracts property from one set of persons in order to give it to another set of persons.

Need-Based Perspectives on Distributive Justice. The moral rationale for specifying need as a relevant criterion for decisions of distributive justice is that a person would be harmed if a need is denied. Put another way, distribution of resources is just when it is based on need; but what is meant by need?

The first distinction to be made is the distinction between all needs and basic or fundamental needs. Distributive justice does not demand that all goods and services be equally distributed for all needs: Not all needs are equally important or fundamental to human survival or flourishment. For example, most persons would not equate the need for jewelry or cosmetics as comparable to the need for adequate oxygen or nutrition. The former two needs are personal needs that are not related to survival, whereas deprivation of the latter two needs can profoundly affect human survival or flourishment.

Thus, within the need-based perspective, the emphasis is on basic or fundamental needs. This is so because basic needs tend to be generic to all humans, and deprivation of these needs can cause serious harm or even death. According to Beauchamp and Childress (1983):

> To say that someone has a "fundamental need" for something is to say that the person will be harmed or detrimentally affected in a fundamental way if that thing is not obtained. Examples of fundamental harms would be malnutrition, serious bodily injury, and the withholding of critical information. Without nutrition, health care, and education, these harms would befall anyone; hence we say we have a fundamental need for such primary goods. (p. 189)

The acceptance of the principle of fundamental needs as a valid material principle of justice commits a provision of whatever is necessary to meet the need. For example, if a nurse administrator works in a state where continuing education is a requirement for continued licensure, then the state must provide opportunities by which this requirement can be met.

Strengths of the need-based perspective include sensitivity to factors over which individuals have no control and accommodation to individual differences and needs. A major problem with the need-based perspective is how to define crucial terms. The concept of needs can be troubling, even if referring to basic needs, because the concept in and of itself may not represent a sufficient basis for a just decision. To illustrate, although two patients may be in serious need of oxygen (an undisputed basic need), nurse administrators may view their equal claims to a new respirator as unfair because one patient's need for oxygen resulted from a serious accident over which the patient had no control, whereas the other patient's need for oxygen resulted from serious neglect to the patient's own health from smoking.

In summary, this overview of four perspectives on distributive justice provides nurse administrators with a basic knowledge base and an organizing framework from which to enhance moral reasoning about distributive justice (*See* Table 3–2). The crux of moral reasoning lies in the ability of nurse administrators to explicitly identify and use ethical principles of distributive justice in decisions in nursing. To this end, two classes of ethical principles were identified: principles of biomedical ethics and material principles of justice.

TABLE 3–2. ETHICAL PRINCIPLES, STRENGTHS, AND POTENTIAL PROBLEMS INHERENT IN FOUR THEORETICAL PERSPECTIVES ON DISTRIBUTIVE JUSTICE

Theoretical Perspective	Strongest Principle of Biomedical Ethics	Examples of Material Principles of Justice	Strengths of Theoretical Perspective	Potential Problems of Theoretical Perspective
Libertarian	Principle of autonomy	To each person according to that person's rights	Commitment to liberty	Unfair to least advantaged members of society
		To each person according to merit	Strong respect for persons	Can lead to inequities in distribution of society's benefits and burdens
		To each person according to societal contribution	Strong respect for individual differences	
Utilitarian	Principle of beneficence	To each person as you would be done to	Strong sense of community	Interests of the majority could override the interests of the minority
		To each person according to the greatest good for the greatest number	Maximizes good for the largest number of people	Individual needs could become subservient to group needs
			Practical approach used in making a decision by assessing consequences	Good and the prevention of harm are not easily quantified
				How the aggregate of societal goods is allocated is not accounted for
Egalitarian	Principles of justice as equality	To each person an equal share	Takes into account the needs of all members of society equally	Not possible to attain equality
		To each person a comparable share	Commitment to democratic principles	Human incentives may be decreased
			Sensitive to the effects of substantial inequalities in the allocation of societal resources	
Need-Based	Principle of nonmaleficence	To each person according to individual needs	Sensitive to factors over which individual has no control	Crucial terms are hard to define
		To each person according to basic needs	Sensitive to individual differences and needs	Difficult to meet commitments if resources are finite or scarce

From: "Ethics, Scarce Resources, and the Nurse Executive" by M. C. Silva, 1984, *Nursing Economic$*, 2, pp. 12–13. Copyright 1984 by Anthony J. Jannetti, Inc., publisher *Nursing Economic$*. Reproduced and modified with permission.

Summary. In this chapter, three major ethical principles are addressed. The first principle, respect for autonomy, means that humans have duties to treat autonomous persons in such a way as to allow them to govern their lives without interference from others. The second principle, beneficence, means that humans have duties to help other persons and not to harm them, including duties to prevent and remove harm or the risk of harm. The third principle, justice, means that persons ought to receive what is due or owed them. With basic ethics terminology defined (Chapter 1), with ethical theories (Chapter 2) and ethical principles (Chapter 3) described, we are now ready in Chapter 4 to address content that underlies ethical decision making.

REFERENCES

American Nurses' Association. (1980). *Nursing: A social policy statement.* Kansas City, MO: Author.

American Nurses' Association. (1985). *Code for nurses with interpretive statements.* Kansas City, MO: Author.

Beauchamp, T. L. (1982a). *Philosophical ethics: An introduction to moral philosophy.* New York: McGraw–Hill.

Beauchamp, T. L. (1982b). Ethical theory and bioethics. In T. L. Beauchamp & L. Walters (Eds.), *Contemporary issues in bioethics* (2nd ed., pp. 1–43). Belmont, CA: Wadsworth.

Beauchamp, T. L., & Childress, J. F. (1983). *Principles of biomedical ethics* (2nd ed.). New York: Oxford University Press.

Beauchamp, T. L., & Pinkard, T. P. (1983). Introduction (part two, justice). In T. L. Beauchamp & T. P. Pinkard (Eds.), *Ethics and public policy: An introduction to ethics* (2nd ed., pp. 128–147). Englewood Cliffs, NJ: Prentice–Hall.

Brock, D. W. (1987). Informed consent. In D. VanDeVeer & T. Regan (Eds.), *Health care ethics: An introduction* (pp. 98–126). Philadelphia: Temple University Press.

Cassileth, B. R., Zupkis, R. V., Sutton-Smith, K., & March, V. (1980). Informed consent—why are its goals imperfectly realized? *The New England Journal of Medicine, 302,* 896–900.

D'Arcy, E. (1963). *Human acts: An essay in their moral evaluation.* Oxford: Clarendon Press.

Downie, R. S., & Telfer, E. (1970). *Respect for persons.* New York: Schocken.

Engelhardt, H. T., Jr. (1986). *The foundations of bioethics.* New York: Oxford University Press.

Faden, R. R., & Beauchamp, T. L. (1986). *A history and theory of informed consent.* New York: Oxford University Press.

Frankena, W. K. (1973). *Ethics* (2nd ed.). Englewood Cliffs, NJ: Prentice–Hall.

International Council of Nurses. (1973). *Code for nurses: Ethical concepts applied to nursing.* Geneva: Author.

Jameton, A. (1984). *Nursing practice: The ethical issues.* Englewood Cliffs, NJ: Prentice–Hall.

Kamen, A. (1987, March 26). Supreme Court upholds affirmative action hiring. *The Washington Post,* pp. A1, A17.

Kant, I. (1981). *Grounding for the metaphysics of morals* (J. W. Ellington, Trans.). Indianapolis: Hackett. (Original work published in German in 1785).

Mill, J. S. (1979). *Utilitarianism* (G. Sher, Ed.). Indianapolis: Hackett. (Original work published 1861)

Muss, H. B., White, D. R., Michielutte, R., Richards, F., II., Cooper, M. R., Williams, S., Stuart, J. J., & Spurr, C. L. (1979). Written informed consent in patients with breast cancer. *Cancer, 43,* 1549–1556.

Rawls, J. (1971). *A theory of justice.* Cambridge, MA: Belknap Press of Harvard University Press.

Silva, M. C. (1984). Ethics, scarce resources, and the nurse executive. *Nursing Economic$, 2,* 11–18.

Silva, M. C. (1985). Comprehension of information for informed consent by spouses of surgical patients. *Research in Nursing and Health, 8,* 117–124.

Veatch, R. M. (1981). *A theory of medical ethics,* New York: Basic Books.

Decision Making, Values, and Stages of Moral Development

Mary Cipriano Silva

Moral courage is a more rare commodity
than bravery in battle or great intelligence.
Robert F. Kennedy

In this chapter, nurse administrators are presented with background knowledge to facilitate ethical decision making. First, theoretical content and practical considerations related to decision making are presented. Next, values, values clarification, and values conflict/resolution are discussed; in addition, present and future values that underlie nursing are addressed. Finally, an overview of moral development is presented.

OVERVIEW OF DECISION MAKING

Prior to discussing the decision making framework formulated in Chapter 5, an overview of decision making is presented. Theoretical approaches to decision making are briefly noted and then practical considerations are discussed.

Theoretical Approaches

For an indepth analysis of theoretical approaches to decision making, see Hammond, McClelland, and Mumpower (1980). These authors discuss six approaches to decision making: decision theory, behavioral decision theory, psychological decision theory, social judgment theory, information integration theory, and attribution theory. From a review of the theories, methods, and procedures underlying these six approaches, the following generalizations can be drawn:

1. Decision making is involved with two complex processes: human judgment and human choice.
2. People do not make decisions in the way predicted by mathematical models of proper decision making because they introduce biases, misinformation, and so forth, into their decision making.
3. Both internal and external factors affect decision making.
4. Unanimity does not exist on how decisions are made or ought to be made.

Therefore, in formulating an ethics decision framework, one must consider both human reasoning and human choice; one must take into account biases that affect decision making; one must be attuned to both internal and external factors that affect decision making; and one must recognize that appropriate decisions can be made in more than one way, with more than one appropriate outcome.

Sources of theoretical materials related to decision making in nursing include Tanner's (1983, pp. 2–32; 1987, pp. 153–173) two reviews of the research literature on clinical judgment and Grier's (1984, pp. 265–287) review of the research literature on information processing. In the former two reviews, Tanner discusses types of decision theory and information processing theory, as well as processes and measures of clinical judgment; in the latter review, Grier focuses on the processing of information for patient care decisions. Readers interested in more detailed theoretical aspects of decision making in nursing should consult these integrative reviews of the literature.

Applied Approaches

Regardless of the decision theory to which one ascribes, ultimately a decision must be made. According to Moody (1983, p. 4), "A *decision* is an action that must be taken when there is no more time for gathering facts." Moody (1983, pp. 7–8) then goes on to discuss five common sense components related to the art of decision making: facts, knowledge, experience, analysis, and judgment.

Facts. One gathers facts to define the boundaries of the problem and to analyze issues intrinsic to it. If facts cannot be obtained, then the decision must be based on available, general information.

Knowledge. One's personal knowledge about a specific problem is useful in clarifying the problem and in selecting a favorable course of action. In the absence of personal knowledge, appropriate consultation can be sought.

Experience. Experience provides one with useful information for solving problems. If an acceptable solution to a problem is found through experience, that solution provides useful guidelines whenever a similar problem arises.

Analysis. Through analysis, one breaks a problem down into its component parts so it can be better understood. Some components of analysis include classification, sequencing, and examination of relationships relevant to the pertinent information.

Judgment. Through judgment, one integrates the preceding facts, knowledge, experience, and results of the analysis. Ideally, this integration leads to a sound decision.

How might these five steps apply to an ethical dilemma in nursing administration? Let us examine the common ethical dilemma of whether patients are competent to make an informed consent decision about their participation in research. Suppose Patient R is hospitalized with breast cancer. The head nurse approaches R to participate in a study on social support and coping with breast cancer. Patient R reads the informed consent form, says she understands it, and signs it. When the head nurse visits R later that day, it is apparent that R is not clear on the study purposes or procedures, yet R insists she wants to participate in the study because she wants to help other women with breast cancer.

Here is an application of Moody's five decision making steps to the preceding situation.

1. **Facts.** Patient R is 75 years old and college educated. She is frequently confined to bed due to the breast cancer. She wants to participate in the study on breast cancer; however, she does not appear to comprehend adequately the information for her informed consent. Thus, R's capacity to give an informed consent is in question.
2. **Knowledge.** The head nurse works on a cancer research unit and is knowledgeable about informed consent. This includes knowing that researchers (e.g., Silva & Sorrell, 1984) have consistently reported a significant and positive relationship between educational level and comprehension; that is, the higher the person's educational level, the greater the person's comprehension of the information for an informed consent. Also that researchers (e.g., Cassileth, Zupkis, Sutton-Smith, & March, 1980; Stanley, Guido, Stanley, & Shortell, 1984) have found that elderly patients and bedridden patients show signifi-

cantly poorer comprehension of information for informed consent than do younger patients and nonbedridden patients. In addition, this head nurse knows that Morrow, Gootnick, and Schmale (1978), in their study with cancer patients, were able to increase comprehension scores in virtually all informed consent areas by allowing patients to take the forms home to read for one to three days.

3. **Experience.** The head nurse has dealt with the problem of questionable competency for an informed consent many times. Experience has shown that, if the patient is not too ill and adequate time is spent with the patient, comprehension can be increased.

4. **Analysis.** Factors operating in Patient R's favor for enhancing her comprehension include her educational level and her desire to participate in the study. Factors operating to inhibit her comprehension include her age and bedridden status. From personal observations of R, the head nurse knows that she is alert and, although frequently confined to bed, is able to take care of many of her activities of daily living. R is also observed to be an avid reader.

5. **Judgment.** Based on the preceding facts, knowledge, experience, and analysis, the head nurse decides to give Patient R the informed consent form to read again, telling her that she can keep the form until she is clear on the information in it. When the head nurse returns several days later to talk to R about the study, she clearly understands the information. Thus, R's wish to participate in the study is granted.

In addition to the preceding five decision making components, Moody (1983, pp. 9–11) discusses several problems that can interfere with a good decision and, thus, should be avoided. Three of these problems are misdirection, bias, and misinterpretation.

Misdirection. Misdirection deals with a proper intent that is erroneously executed. For example, suppose an ethics committee at a local hospital plans to discuss how scarce resources should be allocated among a group of AIDS patients and a group of dialysis patients. During the week the committee is to meet, a nationally recognized expert on AIDS is visiting the community and is asked to participate in the meeting. The committee is intimidated by the expert, however. Thus, although the committee had a proper intent (i.e., to obtain expert advice), the method selected impeded rather than enhanced the committee's goal of discussing an allocation issue.

Bias. As previously noted, people do not make decisions in the way predicted by mathematical models of proper decision making because they introduce biases and misinformation into their thinking. A bias is a factor that prejudices a decision; it is usually an unreasoned and personal distortion of judgment. For example, suppose that among the members of the preceding ethics committee, Member S actively avoids being in the same room with AIDS patients, this avoidance behavior based on fear of contacting AIDS. Member S maintains this stance despite serious efforts made by other committee members to dispel myths regarding the transmission of AIDS. S's bias most likely will affect how S views the care of, and allocation of resources to, the AIDS patients.

Misinterpretation. A third problem that can interfere with a good decision is distortion of data. Such distortion is potentially serious because it can lead to faulty conclusions. A common example is the use of numbers or percents to misrepresent a situation. In keeping with the preceding example, let us suppose that Member S says that 50 percent of the nurses associated with a local health clinic have been infected with the AIDS virus. The percent is correct, but the total number of nurses associated with the clinic is two.

Ideally, the preceding three problems can be diminished by carefully thinking through one's purposes and by being aware of one's biases and how these biases can affect one's own or others' decisions. Awareness of other persons' biases, values, and points of view is important because patient care decisions, including ethics decisions, usually involve more than one person and more than one approach to a problem. Thus, a review of principles related to group decision making is in order.

Moody offers the following ten principles for effective group decision making.

Effective Group Decision Making[1]

1. The group must clearly understand its purpose.
2. The group must be flexible in determining the procedure to be followed to attain its goal.

---

[1]**From:** Moody, P. E. (1983). *Decision making: Proven methods for better decisions.* New York: McGraw–Hill.

3. Group members must communicate freely with one another and understand one another's role.
4. Each member must be committed to the major decisions made after all individual viewpoints have been considered.
5. The group must achieve a balance between individual needs and group productivity.
6. There must be a sharing of group leadership so that all alternatives are equally considered.
7. Group members must feel a high degree of pride in such membership.
8. The group must make good use of the various skills of its members.
9. The group should assess its own progress and take corrective action, if necessary.
10. The group should not be dominated by any one member or the leader. (p. 25)

The preceding group could be comprised of only two persons (e.g., nurse and doctor; patient and nurse; patient and doctor) or a larger number of persons (e.g., an institutional ethics committee; a multidisciplinary team conference). Regardless of number, the ten principles help group members to function in a manner conducive to the give-and-take necessary in making health care decisions, including ethics decisions.

In summary, then, how does the preceding background knowledge about decision making affect ethical decision making? First, because decision making is affected by internal factors such as values and external factors such as agency policies, it is a complex process; consequently, unanimity does not always exist on how decisions (including ethics decisions) are made or ought to be made. Second, since decision making is a process, the process can be made somewhat explicit. This explicitness allows the analysis of ethical dilemmas to proceed in a reasonably systematic manner, as we shall see in Chapter 5. Third, since most decisions in health care and in health care ethics occur within the give-and-take of a group, it is helpful to apply principles of group dynamics to decision making. One important area of give-and-take in health care ethics involves attending to other persons' values. It is to this topic that we now turn.

OVERVIEW OF VALUES

Definitions

Values guide behavior; they are enduring ideals or beliefs to which a person is committed (American Association of Colleges of Nursing, 1986, p. 5). According to Steele & Harmon (1983, pp. 1–13), values originate from one's life experiences and contribute to the integration of one's personality. Values reflect a person's enduring beliefs that some stances are preferable to other stances and, as such, become a standard for guiding one's actions.

Value Neutrality. A term commonly associated with values is *value neutrality*, which refers to the position that "no matter what values the professional holds, he or she must remain neutral relative to the values of the care recipient" (Wright, 1987, p. 15). There are pros and cons to this position. On the pro side, it is argued that the care recipient has a right to his or her values and that the professional should not interfere with these values. On the con side, it is argued that the preceding position is untenable because it is not always possible or desirable for a professional to remain neutral about the values of the care recipient, especially when the care recipient's values involve harm to self or others. That is, there are times when, within the view of most professionals or society, a person's values should not be supported because they are destructive and arguably wrong. In this situation the professional has an obligation to persuade the person to rethink the values. To not recognize this situation could lead to failure of one's professional responsibilities. According to Wright (1987),

> Value neutrality is really nothing more than an excuse to not deal with ethical problems and to avoid facing the real problems of the world. Instead of an ethical rule, the call for value neutrality is more reasonably understood as a request for tolerance and recognition that there are acceptable alternatives to *some* of one's own values. That, however, does not lead to the conclusion that the correctness of moral judgments is solely a matter of unquestionable individual preference. What does follow is that we have an obligation to consider the reasons supporting adherence to certain values, consideration which may lead to either acceptance or rejection of those values. (p. 16)

Values Clarification. Interest in values clarification came about in response to the inadequacies of earlier methods of values instruction that either focused on an abandonment of inculcating values or on an indoctrination of them (Brummer, 1984). According to Steele and Harmon (1983),

> Values clarification fosters the making of choices and facilitates decision-making. It is a process of discovery and allows the person to discover through feelings and analysis of behavior what choices to make when alternatives are presented, and to identify whether or not these choices are rationally made or are the result of previous conditioning. The values clarification process attempts to bring to conscious awareness the values and underlying motivations that guide one's actions. (p. 13)

Brummer (1984) identifies the following premises underlying values clarification:

1. Clarification of one's values is important and can occur through a self-examination process.
2. This process, known as values clarification, aims at values discernment and formulation, *not* at values inculcation.
3. The preceding discernment and formulation is arrived at through discovery and reflective judgment in arriving at certain universally valid values.
4. In situations of value conflict, most persons can be trusted to choose wisely if they follow the preceding reflective process in a nonthreatening atmosphere.

Although the preceding premises are somewhat controversial, they are included herein because of the importance of values clarification to the analysis and resolution of ethical dilemmas.

Value Conflicts. In health care situations, however, focusing on one's own values through values clarification is often not enough; one must also be sensitive to the values of others, especially in situations where values conflict. In value conflicts, a tension may exist among one's own values and the values of others, causing difficulties in the resolution of ethical dilemmas. These difficulties may take the following forms: (1) uncertainty over whose values should take precedence, and (2) inability to make a decision.

There is little in the health care literature about *how* to analyze and resolve value conflicts related to ethics; consequently, the following guidelines are proposed. The first set of guidelines focuses on the analysis of value conflicts. The analysis occurs through reflection on the following set of questions:

1. *Persons holding the values:* What persons are most involved in the resolution of the ethics value conflict?
2. *Nature of the values:* What values relevant to the ethics conflict are operating among the most involved persons?
3. *Strength of the values:* What is the strength of the values held by persons involved in the ethics conflict?
4. *Congruency of the values:* Which of the preceding values are most congruent with professional practice and patient well-being?
5. *Outcome of the values:* Who will be most affected by the underlying values that affect the ethics decision? How will these persons be affected?

Based on the preceding assessment, a second set of guidelines are proposed for the resolution of ethical value conflicts. These guidelines serve as organizing principles for action.

1. Values that support ethical professional practice and patient well-being should take priority over those that do not.
2. Stronger values that support ethical professional practice and patient well-being should generally take precedence over weaker values that support ethical professional practice and patient well-being.
3. All things considered, values of persons who will be most affected by the decision should take precedence over values of persons who will be less affected by the decision.

Values Underlying the Profession

As the preceding guidelines emphasize, values that support professional practice and patient well-being merit high priority. But what are these values? Two recent reports (American Association of Colleges of Nursing, 1986; Center for Nursing Excellence, 1987) give some insight into current values that underlie the nursing profession.

The report from the AACN focuses on the essentials of college and university education for professional nursing, both now and in the future. A national panel was selected "to define the essential knowledge, practice, and values for the education of the professional nurse. . ." (AACN, 1986, p. iii). Over 25,000 copies of a working document were given to members of the nursing, health care, and higher education professions. Open hearings followed in seven locations across the country. In addition, nearly 1500 persons responded in writing to the document.

Based on the preceding data, the panel recommended the following seven values as essential for professional nursing.

1. *Altruism:* Concern for the welfare of others.
2. *Equality:* Having the same rights, privileges, or status.
3. *Esthetics:* Qualities of objects, events, and persons that provide satisfaction.
4. *Freedom:* Capacity to exercise choice.
5. *Human Dignity:* Inherent worth and uniqueness of an individual.
6. *Justice:* Upholding moral and legal principles.
7. *Truth:* Faithfulness to fact or reality. (AACN, 1986, pp. 6–7)

The panel then went on to state that, within specific decision making contexts, the professional nurse assigns priorities to these values. The nurse's goal is to provide patients with safe and humanistic care that focuses on health and quality of life.

The report of the Center for Nursing Excellence is an Executive Summary that focuses on the future of hospital-based nursing in the years 2000 and 2020. Using Delphi survey techniques, data within the report were collected from nurse leaders with expertise in administration, education, and practice, as well as from persons with knowledge in health care trends and futures research methodology. Four dominant themes/values emerged:

1. *Altruism:* Nurses will continue to reaffirm their commitment to humanistic care for people.
2. *Patient Rights:* Nurses will continue to educate and counsel patients and will support patients' rights in controlling life. They also will align with consumers and patients to advocate on their behalf.
3. *Autonomy:* Nurses will continue to strive for autonomy in practice, education, and policy decisions. This striving will continue despite a sense of powerlessness.
4. *New Opportunities:* Nurses will seek new opportunities in wellness and occupational health. In addition, nurses will seek new opportunities in the roles of entrepreneur and health care broker. (Center for Nursing Excellence, 1987)

Taken together, these two reports provide insight into the present and a glimpse into the future of what nurses value. For a more detailed assessment of values and nursing, however, let us examine three current research studies.

Values and Ethics: Examples of Nursing Research

Three recent examples of nursing research that focus on values and ethics in nursing are summarized. Gortner, Hudes, and Zyzanski (1984) measured values in the choice of treatment for coronary artery disease. Based on a pilot study, they formulated two hypotheses:

   I. Individual and family values will be positively related in both surgical and medical treatment situations; correlations will remain consistent over time upon retest of the surgical treatment group.
  II. There will be no difference among treatment groups in the values of Autonomy, Beneficence/Nonmaleficence, and Justice. (p. 320)

Sample 1 was composed of 70 surgical patients who underwent a first coronary artery bypass grafting and their families; sample 2 was composed of 30 medical patients under treatment for coronary artery disease and their families. The Gortner Values in the Choice of Treatment Inventory was administered to the preceding 100 patients and to one of their family members (usually the spouse) at the initial interview and at one month after discharge (for the bypass patients).

Both Hypothesis I and II were supported. Regarding Hypothesis I, the investigators found a significant (albeit weak) correlation between patient/spouse surgical pairs on the overall values of autonomy, beneficence, and justice. The strongest patient/spouse correlation was for beneficence. Regarding Hypothesis II, the investigators found no significant interactions or significant differences by patient or spouse status, or by location. The differences in scales were highly significant, however; that is, patients and spouses valued autonomy more highly than beneficence, and they valued beneficence more highly than justice.

Within the framework of this study, two implications for nursing practice are: (1) If nurses know the moral values of the patient, they also can predict (albeit weakly) the moral values of the family; and (b) if patients and families place a higher value on autonomy than on beneficence or justice, some conflicts between nurses and patients/families may occur because of the traditional emphasis in nursing on beneficence. If the predictions of the Center for Nursing Excellence discussed in the preceding section are correct, however, patients' and nurses' values about autonomy may be more congruent by the years 2000 and 2020.

In a second study, Ketefian (1985) investigated the relationship

between bureaucratic and professional role conceptions and moral behavior. Role conception was measured by scores on two subscales of
the Nursing Role Conception instrument: the bureaucratic and the professional subscales. For each subscale, a normative, a categorical, and a
discrepancy score was obtained.

The instrument consisted of six stories involving nurses in ethical
dilemmas. A list of several nursing actions followed each story. The
respondent was to decide: (1) whether the nurse facing the dilemma
should or should not engage in each nursing action (A scores), and (2)
whether the nurse facing the dilemma is likely to engage in each nursing action (B scores). Moral behavior was measured by the column B
scores on the Judgments About Nursing Decisions instrument. Each
appropriate nursing action received a score of 1; each inappropriate
action received a score of 0. These numbers were added to yield a total
score on moral behavior.

Several hypotheses were formulated that focused on how nurses'
professional–bureaucratic role conceptions and their perceptions of the
discrepancy between actual values and ideal values affected the way
they made judgments about nursing actions related to moral behavior.
Results were as follows:

1. The professional categorical role conception and moral behavior
   were found to be positively related, whereas both the professional role discrepancy and the professional normative role conception were found to be negatively related to moral behavior.
2. Bureaucratic role discrepancy and moral behavior were found to
   be positively related.
3. Combinations of the various role conceptions (e.g., professional
   and bureaucratic role discrepancies, professional categorical
   and bureaucratic categorical role conceptions, and professional
   normative and bureaucratic normative role conceptions) ac-
   counted for greater variance in moral behavior than either one
   of the pairs of variables alone.

Within the framework of this study the implications for nursing
practice are: (1) If nurse administrators can determine nurse employees'
conceptions of their role, they may be able to predict professional values such as moral attitudes; and (2) nurse executives must recognize
that role conceptualization as it relates to moral behavior is complex.

In a third study, Swider, McElmurry, and Yarling (1985) studied
the decision making process used by 775 senior baccalaureate nursing
students (146 small groups) in resolving a hypothetical ethical dilemma

in which a drug error that killed a patient was being covered up by the attending physician. Each of the 146 groups was asked to read the case and decide what steps the nurse should take to resolve the dilemma. The groups were to record the first step and all subsequent steps until they had exhausted all reasonable steps the nurse should take. Persons who disagreed with the group decision were asked to write a minority report.

Of the 1163 decisions made by the groups, 9 percent were classified as patient-centered, 19 percent were classified as physician-centered, 60 percent were classified as bureaucracy-centered, and 12 percent were classified as other. Of the 107 decisions made by students in 15 groups submitting minority reports, 10 percent were classified as patient-centered, 58 percent were classified as bureaucracy-centered, 18 percent were classified as physician-centered, and 14 percent were classified as other. When the first and last decisions in each group were assessed, the following trend emerged: First decisions tended to be bureaucracy-centered (89 percent), whereas last decisions tended to be a mix of patient-centered (29 percent), physician-centered (14 percent), bureaucracy-centered (27 percent), and other (29 percent).

An implication for nursing practice is as follows: One can predict that the dominant underlying value of student nurses in terms of initial and overall ethical decision making will be bureaucracy-centered. Although at first glance this seems to conflict with the nurse's role as patient advocate, one can conjecture reasons for bureaucratic responses, particularly with the first decision. For example, it does not seem unreasonable for a nurse to want to file an incident report (classified as a bureaucracy-centered response) before discussing the problem with the family (classified as a patient-oriented response).

In summary, then, how does knowledge about values, and research on values, affect ethical decision making? First, knowledge about values, and research on values, helps one to understand their pervasiveness and complexity in decision making. Second, because values are enduring beliefs, one cannot expect persons to give them up lightly when faced with opposing beliefs in decision making. Of course enduring does not necessarily mean a logical, correct, or morally justifiable belief; hence, these latter characteristics provide some rationale for overriding questionable values when a decision must be made. Third, values clarification as a part of the decision making process helps one to assess whether a value is appropriate for a given ethical dilemma or whether the value may need modification in light of new evidence.

One type of new evidence related to values is how men and women vary in their moral development. This topic, as well as others related to moral development, is discussed in the following section.

OVERVIEW OF MORAL DEVELOPMENT

The decisions one makes regarding an ethical dilemma can be influenced by one's level of moral development. According to Omery (1983), there are three dominant models of moral development: psychoanalytic, social learning, and cognitive developmental models. Although cognitive developmental is the dominant model of moral development presented in the nursing literature, the other two are addressed briefly as a basis of comparison. The nurse administrator must be aware, however, that aspects of all three models are open to question; therefore, the models and the assumptions underlying them must not be accepted unquestioningly.

Psychoanalytic Models

According to Omery's interpretation of psychoanalytic models, the human personality is divided into three structures: id, ego, and superego. Moral development is associated with the superego and occurs from the resolution of the Oedipus complex and castration anxiety. As part of the process of resolution, both males and females (for different reasons) identify with the father and introject his value system. In classic psychoanalytic theory, the male develops a differentiated superego, whereas the female develops a poorly differentiated one. According to Omery, however, results of empirical research on psychoanalytic models have been questionable or not supported.

Social Learning Model

Omery's interpretation and assessment of social learning models are discussed in the following paragraphs. In social learning theory, moral behavior (as all behavior) is learned from observing how others behave. Moral development represents a process where specific competencies such as cognitive capabilities are learned and actively stored as potential behaviors. The activation of these potential behaviors depends on: (1) an individual's expectation that a particular reinforcement will occur, (2) the degree of an individual's preference for that reinforcement, and (3) contingency rules which guide an individual's behavior in the absence of (or in spite of) the reinforcement(s).

In the social learning model of moral development, the transition from child to adult morality follows a sequence. First, control is externally provided by adults who take measures to prevent the child from harm. Second, as the child matures physical sanctions are replaced by social ones, and external sanctions are gradually replaced by internal controls. Third, there is a shift in focus from assessing the morality of individual acts to assessing the moral implications of the individual acts in terms of society.

Empirical research on social learning models has been limited and has focused primarily on the role of modeling or observation in the learning experience that constitutes moral development. Investigators have found that modeling of others is most likely to occur when a model acts on (rather than verbalizes or writes about) a commitment and when the model is viewed as competent and nurturing. Overall, the methodologies of these studies are sound; however, the relationship of the social learning model to the rest of the study often is ambiguous.

Cognitive Developmental Models

The cognitive developmental model best known to nurses is the one developed by Kohlberg (1976; 1981). Kohlberg's work is an outgrowth of Piaget's view of justice as the core of morality. Kohlberg, however, replaced Piaget's two-stage model with a three-level one that contained two stages at each level, as shown in the following.

The Six Stages of Moral Judgment[2]

Level A. Preconventional Level

Stage 1. The Stage of Punishment and Obedience

Content. Right is literal obedience to rules and authority, avoiding punishment, and not doing physical harm.

1. What is right is to avoid breaking rules, to obey for obedience' sake, and to avoid doing physical damage to people and property.

---

[2]**From:** Kohlberg, L. (1981). *Essays on moral development: Vol. 1. The philosophy of moral development: Moral stages and the idea of justice* (pp. 409–412). San Francisco: Harper & Row. Excerpt from *The Philosophy of Moral Development* by Lawrence Kohlberg, © 1981 by Lawrence Kohlberg. Reprinted by permission of Harper & Row, Publishers, Inc.

2. The reasons for doing right are avoidance of punishment and the superior power of authorities.

Social Perspective. This stage takes an egocentric point of view. A person at this stage doesn't consider the interests of others or recognize they differ from actor's, and doesn't relate two points of view. Actions are judged in terms of physical consequences rather than in terms of psychological interests of others. Authority's perspective is confused with one's own.

Stage 2. The Stage of Individual Instrumental Purpose and Exchange

Content. Right is serving one's own or other's [sic] needs and making fair deals in terms of concrete exchange.

1. What is right is following rules when it is to someone's immediate interest. Right is acting to meet one's own interests and needs and letting others do the same. Right is also what is fair; that is, what is an equal exchange, a deal, an agreement.
2. The reason for doing right is to serve one's own needs or interests in a world where one must recognize that other people have their interests, too.

Social Perspective. This stage takes a concrete individualistic perspective. A person at this stage separates own interests and points of view from those of authorities and others. He or she is aware everybody has individual interests to pursue and these conflict, so that right is relative (in the concrete individualistic sense). The person integrates or relates conflicting individual interests to one another through instrumental exchange of services, through instrumental need for the other and the other's goodwill, or through fairness giving each person the same amount.

Level B. Conventional Level

Stage 3. The Stage of Mutual Interpersonal Expectations, Relationships, and Conformity

Content. The right is playing a good (nice) role, being concerned about the other people and their feelings, keeping loyalty and trust with partners, and being motivated to follow rules and expectations.

1. What is right is living up to what is expected by people close to one or what people generally expect of people in one's role as son, sister, friend, and so on. "Being good" is important and means having good motives, showing concern about others. It also means keeping mutual relationships, maintaining trust, loyalty, respect, and gratitude.
2. Reasons for doing right are needing to be good in one's own eyes and those of others, caring for others, and because if one puts oneself in the other person's place one would want good behavior from the self (Golden Rule).

Social Perspective. This stage takes the perspective of the individual in relationship to other individuals. A person at this stage is aware of shared feelings, agreements, and expectations, which take primacy over individual interests. The person relates points of view through the "concrete Golden Rule," putting oneself in the other person's shoes. He or she does not consider generalized "system" perspective.

Stage 4. The Stage of Social System and Conscience Maintenance

Content. The right is doing one's duty in society, upholding the social order, and maintaining the welfare of society or the group.

1. What is right is fulfilling the actual duties to which one has agreed. Laws are to be upheld except in extreme cases where they conflict with other fixed social duties and rights. Right is also contributing to society, the group, or institution.
2. The reasons for doing right are to keep the institution going as a whole, self-respect or conscience as meeting one's defined obligations, or the consequences: "What if everyone did it?"

Social Perspective. This stage differentiates societal point of view from interpersonal agreement or motives. A person at this stage takes the viewpoint of the system, which defines roles and rules. He or she considers individual relations in terms of place in the system.

Level B/C. Transitional Level

This level is postconventional but not yet principled.

Content of Transition. At Stage 4½, choice is personal and subjective.

It is based on emotions, conscience is seen as arbitrary and relative, as are ideas such as "duty" and "morally right."

Transitional Social Perspective. At this stage, the perspective is that of an individual standing outside of his own society and considering himself as an individual making decisions without a generalized commitment or contract with society. One can pick and choose obligations, which are defined by particular societies, but one has no principles for such choice.

Level C. Postconventional and Principled Level

Moral decisions are generated from rights, values, or principles that are (or could be) agreeable to all individuals composing or creating a society designed to have fair and beneficial practices.

Stage 5. The Stage of Prior Rights and Social Contract or Utility

Content. The right is upholding the basic rights, values, and legal contracts of a society, even when they conflict with the concrete rules and laws of the group.

1. What is right is being aware of the fact that people hold a variety of values and opinions, that most values and rules are relative to one's group. These "relative" rules should usually be upheld, however, in the interest of impartiality and because they are the social contract. Some nonrelative values and rights such as life, and liberty, however, must be upheld in any society and regardless of majority opinion.
2. Reasons for doing right are, in general, feeling obligated to obey the law because one has made a social contract to make and abide by laws for the good of all and to protect their own rights and the rights of others. Family, friendship, trust, and work obligations are also commitments or contracts freely entered into and entail respect for the rights of others. One is concerned that laws and duties be based on rational calculation of overall utility: "the greatest good for the greatest number."

Social Perspective. This stage takes a prior-to-society perspective—that of a rational individual aware of values and rights prior to social attachments and contracts. The person integrates perspectives by formal mechanisms of agreement, contract, objective impartiality, and due process. He or she considers the moral point of view and the legal point of view, recognizes they conflict, and finds it difficult to integrate them.

Stage 6. The Stage of Universal Ethical Principles

Content. This stage assumes guidance by universal ethical principles that all humanity should follow.

1. Regarding what is right, Stage 6 is guided by universal ethical principles. Particular laws or social agreements are usually valid because they rest on such principles. When laws violate these principles, one acts in accordance with the principle. Principles are universal principles of justice: the equality of human rights and respect for the dignity of human beings as individuals. These are not merely values that are recognized, but are also principles used to generate particular decisions.
2. The reason for doing right is that, as a rational person, one has seen the validity of principles and has become committed to them.

Social Perspective. This stage takes the perspective of a moral point of view from which social arrangements derive or on which they are grounded. The perspective is that of any rational individual recognizing the nature of morality or the basic moral premise of respect for other persons as ends, not means.

Kohlberg's work is controversial because of his assertion that most females do not proceed in moral development beyond Level II, Stage B. Gilligan (1977; 1979; 1982) has disputed Kohlberg's work, arguing that female moral development is different from male moral development. According to Gilligan, this difference results from how men and women engage in social interactions. Women, because of their traditional powerlessness, have coped by developing a sense of responsibility based on caring rather than on individual rights (typical of men). Gilligan's levels of moral development are outlined in the following paragraph; however, keep in mind that Gilligan's model also has been criticized. One criticism is that the model too sharply dichotomizes the behavior of men and women (Thompson & Thompson, 1985, pp. 65–68); another criticism is that Gilligan's work has not been successfully replicated.

Levels of Women's Moral Judgment[3]

Level I: Orientation to Individual Survival. At level one the self is the sole object of concern and the primary concern is that of survival. The self is constrained by powerlessness. Morality is viewed as sanctions imposed by society.

The First Transition: From Selfishness to Responsibility. In the first transition, there is a reappraisal of self-interest and a movement toward connection or attachment to others. In this transition there is a move from selfishness toward responsibility.

Level II: Goodness as Self-Sacrifice. Moral judgment is viewed as shared expectations and norms. Survival depends on acceptance by others. Good is equated with caring for, protecting, and not hurting others, with insufficient consideration of this self-sacrifice to self. Thus, mutual care and dependence are intertwined.

The Second Transition: From Goodness to Truth. In the second transition, self-sacrifice in the service of a morality of care is questioned. Thus, the issue of responsibility to self, as well as to others, is raised in an effort to reconcile the disparity between care and hurt. A new judgment emerges whose first demand is honesty to self and whose criterion is a shift from goodness to truth.

Level III: The Morality of Nonviolence. In level three, there is an awareness of the moral and psychological necessity for an equation of worth between self and others, an equation that leaves both self and others intact. There is a willingness to express and take responsibility for one's actions through a responsibility of care for self and others. The obligation not to hurt or exploit self and others serves as a universal guide to moral choice. The morality of responsibility (rather than the morality of rights) underlies this highest stage of moral judgment.

---

[3]**From:** Gilligan, C. (1977). In a different voice: Women's conceptions of self and of morality. *Harvard Educational Review, 47,* 481–517.

The Cognitive Developmental Model: Examples of Nursing Research

Results of empirical research based on Kohlberg's cognitive developmental model have been debatable, with some studies supporting and other studies refuting the model (Omery, 1983). Issues surrounding testing of the model include whether young adults regress at the model's higher stages, whether the model is universal to all persons regardless of religion or culture, whether the tool used to collect the data is valid, and whether moral stages and moral behaviors are positively correlated. Despite these concerns, there is sufficient empirical support for Kohlberg's model to consider its use in nursing.

Several nurse investigators have used the model as a theoretical basis for research. Crisham's (1981) primary purpose was to investigate the difference between nurses' responses to hypothetical moral dilemmas and their responses to real-life nursing dilemmas. The sample of 225 was composed of five subject groups: staff nurses with associate degrees in nursing (N=57), staff nurses with baccalaureate degrees in nursing (N=85), master's degree expert nurses (N=10), college junior prenurses (N=36), and graduate level nonnurses (N=37).

The Nursing Dilemma Test (NDT) was developed to measure nurses' responses to recurrent nursing dilemmas. The final NDT consisted of six recurrent ethical dilemmas in clinical practice. For each dilemma, the research subject was asked to respond to three tasks: (1) decide what the nurse should do; (2) rank, in order of importance, the moral and practical aspects of six considerations; and (3) note the degree of previous involvement with a similar nursing dilemma.

Results were as follows:

1. There was a low, but significantly positive, correlation between subjects' moral judgment about hypothetical general dilemmas and about real-life nursing dilemmas.
2. Subjects who had encountered similar moral dilemmas scored significantly higher on indexes reflecting principled thinking than those who had not encountered the dilemma.
3. Overall, the higher the level of education, the higher the indexes that reflected principled thinking.
4. Mean scores for practical considerations did not differ significantly across the five groups. When experience was considered, however, the more-experienced nurses had significantly higher scores on practical considerations than the less-experienced nurses. On the other hand, the more-experienced nurses tended not to have the higher moral judgment scores.

5. There was no consistent pattern in hypothetical and nursing moral judgment scores of staff nurses with less than one year of clinical experience and those with more than five years of clinical experience.

These results suggest that principled moral reasoning may be enhanced through higher education (particularly at the master's level) and through repeated exposures to a moral dilemma. In addition, the potential tension between practical considerations and principled moral judgment was raised, that is, higher practical consideration scores were not associated with higher moral judgment scores.

In a second study also using Kohlberg's levels and stages of moral development as a theoretical rationale for her study, Ketefian (1981) studied the relationship among critical thinking, educational preparation, and development of moral judgment among 79 practicing registered nurses. Critical thinking was measured by the Critical Thinking Appraisal Test Form ZM, moral reasoning by the Defining Issues Test; and type of educational program categorized into professional (a baccalaureate or higher degree) and technical (an associate degree or diploma).

Results were as follows:

1. There was a significant and positive relationship between critical thinking and moral reasoning.
2. There was a significant difference in moral reasoning between professional and technical nurses, with professional nurses displaying more advanced levels of moral reasoning.
3. Educational preparation and critical thinking taken together predicted greater variance in moral reasoning than when either variable was considered separately.

In a third study, Reid-Priest (1984) assessed the moral reasoning process of critical care nurses. Although Reid-Priest used Kohlberg's theory of cognitive development as one of her theoretical frameworks, she made a special point of discussing the gender limitations of Kohlberg's model (i.e., the fact that the model was developed from male-dominated research). She then mentioned Gilligan's model as an alternative to Kohlberg's because of Gilligan's focus on women's development.

Reid-Priest's sample included 103 nurses from 11 critical care units in three facilities. Moral reasoning was measured by the Defining Issues Test and the Nursing Dilemma Test. She formulated six hypotheses to determine the relationship of position, length of clinical experience, and education on moral judgment as measured by scores on the two preceding tests. Her results: Level of education was positively related to moral judgment while position and length of clinical experience were not related significantly to moral judgment.

The results of this study, like the two preceding ones, emphasize that level of education is important to level of moral reasoning, with higher levels of education facilitating moral reasoning. The studies do not, however, establish whether there is a relationship between moral reasoning and moral/ethical behavior.

Based on the preceding studies, how does knowledge of moral development and reasoning facilitate ethical decision making? First, investigators have begun to validate that moral development can be learned. Second, they have begun to validate that moral reasoning can be enhanced through increased education, increased critical thinking, and repeated exposure to an ethical dilemma. Therefore, the background that a nurse administrator brings to an ethics decision-making situation may affect the quality of moral reasoning.

Summary. In this chapter, background knowledge pertinent to ethical decision making is discussed. From this background knowledge and research, several generalizations about decision making, values, and moral development emerge:

1. Unlike mathematical models of proper decision making, people introduce biases and misinformation into their decision making.
2. Both internal and external factors affect decision making.
3. There is lack of agreement on how decisions ought to be made or are made.
4. Decision making is a process; therefore, one can often use the process in analyzing ethical dilemmas.
5. Since most decisions involving ethics occur in a group, effective group decision making is important in facilitating resolution of ethical dilemmas.
6. Values can be better understood through values clarification.
7. Value conflicts occur frequently in the process of resolving ethical dilemmas; thus, conflict analysis and resolution is pertinent to ethical decision making.
8. Moral development is a process that can be learned.
9. Moral reasoning can be enhanced through increased education, increased critical thinking, and repeated exposures to an ethical dilemma.

What, then, can we conclude from the information in this chapter? We can conclude that a variety of background knowledge (e.g., decision theory, group process, stages of moral development) is needed to maximize effective decision making. In addition, nurse administrators' level of education (baccalaureate or higher) and their past experience with resolving ethical dilemmas can facilitate effective ethical decision making. With this groundwork laid, we now turn our attention in Chapter 5 to an ethics decision framework.

REFERENCES

American Association of Colleges of Nursing. (1986). *Essentials of college and university education for professional nursing: Final report.* Washington, DC: Author.

Brummer, J. J. (1984). Moralizing and the philosophy of value education. *Educational Forum, 3,* 263–275.

Cassileth, B. R., Zupkis, R. V., Sutton-Smith, K., & March, V. (1980). Informed consent—Why are its goals imperfectly realized? *New England Journal of Medicine, 302,* 896–900.

Center for Nursing Excellence. (1987). *Nursing 2020: A study of the future of hospital-based nursing. Executive summary.* Los Angeles: Author.

Crisham, P. (1981). Measuring moral judgment in nursing dilemmas. *Nursing Research, 30,* 104–110.

Gilligan, C. (1977). In a different voice: Women's conceptions of self and of morality. *Harvard Educational Review, 47,* 481–517.

Gilligan, C. (1979). Woman's place in man's life cycle. *Harvard Educational Review, 49,* 431–446.

Gilligan, C. (1982). *In a different voice: Psychological theory and women's development.* Cambridge, MA: Harvard University Press.

Gortner, S. R., Hudes, M., & Zyzanski, S. J. (1984). Appraisal of values in the choice of treatment. *Nursing Research, 33,* 319–324.

Grier, M. R. (1984). Information processing in nursing practice. In H. H. Werley & J. J. Fitzpatrick (Eds.), *Annual review of nursing research* (Vol. 2, pp. 265–287). New York: Springer.

Hammond, K. R., McClelland, G. H., & Mumpower, J. (1980). *Human judgment and decision making: Theories, methods, and procedures.* New York: Praeger.

Ketefian, S. (1981). Critical thinking, educational preparation, and development of moral judgment among selected groups of practicing nurses. *Nursing Research, 30,* 98–103.

Ketefian, S. (1985). Professional and bureaucratic role conceptions and moral behavior among nurses. *Nursing Research, 34,* 248–253.

Kohlberg, L. (1976). Moral stages and moralization: The cognitive-developmental approach. In T. Lickona (Ed.), *Moral development and behavior: Theory, research, and social issues* (pp. 31–53). New York: Holt, Rinehart & Winston.

Kohlberg, L. (1981). *Essays on moral development: Vol. 1. The philosophy of moral development: Moral stages and the idea of justice* (pp. 409–412). San Francisco: Harper & Row.

Moody, P. E. (1983). *Decision making: Proven methods for better decisions.* New York: McGraw–Hill.

Morrow, G., Gootnick, J., & Schmale, A. (1978). A simple technique for increasing cancer patients' knowledge of informed consent to treatment. *Cancer, 42,* 793–799.

Omery, A. (1983). Moral development: A differential evaluation of dominant models. *Advances in Nursing Science, 6*(1), 1–17.

Reid-Priest, A. (1984). The moral reasoning process of critical care nurses. *Virginia Nurse, 52,* 68.

Silva, M. C., & Sorrell, J. M. (1984). Factors influencing comprehension of information for informed consent: Ethical implications for nursing research. *International Journal of Nursing Studies, 21,* 233–240.

Stanley, B., Guido, J., Stanley, M., & Shortell, D. (1984). The elderly patient and informed consent: Empirical findings. *Journal of the American Medical Association, 252,* 1302–1306.

Steele, S. M., & Harmon, V. M. (1983). *Values clarification in nursing* (2nd ed.). Norwalk, CT: Appleton–Century–Crofts.

Swider, S. M., McElmurry, B. J., & Yarling, R. R. (1985). Ethical decision making in a bureaucratic context by senior nursing students. *Nursing Research, 34,* 108–112.

Tanner, C. A. (1983). Research on clinical judgment. In W. L. Holzemer (Ed.), *Review of research in nursing education* (pp. 2–32). Thorofare, NJ: Slack.

Tanner, C. A. (1987). Teaching clinical judgment. In J. J. Fitzpatrick & R. L. Taunton (Eds.). *Annual review of nursing research* (Vol. 5, pp. 153–173). New York: Springer.

Thompson, J. E., & Thompson, H. O. (1985). *Bioethical decision making for nurses.* Norwalk, CT: Appleton–Century–Crofts.

Wright, R. A. (1987). *Human values in health care: The practice of ethics.* New York: McGraw–Hill.

PART II

Application

Part II of this book contains an ethics decision framework, presented in Chapter 5; this framework serves to organize the content in Chapters 6 through 8. The framework is formative and, thus, in a state of evolution. Due to its formative nature, the framework does not (nor is it intended to) encompass all components needed to analyze every ethical dilemma in nursing administration. Rather, it is a starting point from which components can be added or deleted as necessary.

For consistency in Part II, conflicts between ethical principles are highlighted. In Chapter 6, conflicts between the ethical principle of autonomy and the ethical principle of beneficence are examined. In Chapter 7, conflicts between the ethical principle of beneficence and the ethical principle of nonmaleficence are examined. In Chapter 8, conflicts between the ethical principle of justice and the ethical principle of beneficence are examined.

Not all conflicts in ethics are between or among ethical principles. Conflicts may also occur, for example, between rights and/or duties and/or role obligations. In any given patient situation, several ethical conflicts may emerge. An ethics decision framework such as that described in Chapter 5 helps to sort out these conflicts.

All six cases presented in Chapters 6 through 8 are real; they were actually encountered by the nurse administrators who wrote the cases. Using the framework described in Chapter 5, the six cases were analyzed by three colleague contributors and the author. The framework fits some of the cases better than others, underscoring the formative nature of the framework.

Once the cases were analyzed, the analyses were commented upon by the nurse administrators who wrote the cases. This gave each nurse administrator a retrospective opportunity to reflect upon the case she had written.

In addition to the cases presented in Chapters 6 through 8, six additional cases are presented in Appendix B. In total, 12 cases are presented in this book. The cases were carefully selected to represent ethical issues faced by today's nurse administrators.

5

Ethics Decision Framework

Mary Cipriano Silva

Thought is the strongest thing we have.
Work done by true and profound thought—
that is real force.
Albert Schweitzer

This chapter sets the stage for the remainder of the book. The decision making framework conceptualized herein is used to analyze the administrative ethical dilemmas in Chapters 6 through 8. Here five criteria relevant to the conceptualization of an ethics decision framework are identified. Examples of several ethics decision frameworks used in health care are summarized. Drawing from components of these frameworks, the following five-part ethics decision framework is then presented.

Ethics Decision Framework

I. Data Collection and Assessment
  A. Situational Considerations
  B. Health Team Considerations
  C. Organizational Considerations
II. Problem Identification
  A. Ethical Considerations
  B. Nonethical Considerations
III. Consideration of Possible Actions
  A. Utilitarian Thinking
  B. Deontological Thinking
IV. Decision and Selection of Course of Action
  A. Contribution of Internal/Group Factors
  B. Contribution of External Factors
  C. Quality of Decision and Course of Action
V. Reflection on Decision and Course of Action
  A. Reflection on Decision
  B. Reflection on Course of Action

CRITERIA FOR ETHICS
DECISION FRAMEWORK

The decision framework formulated in this chapter was conceptualized to meet the following five criteria:

1. *Adequacy:* The framework focuses on content relevant to ethics and ethical dilemmas instead of other types of content.
2. *Consistency:* Use of the framework on more than one occasion yields the same or similar outcomes in similar situations.
3. *Coherence:* Components of the framework are internally consistent and logical.
4. *Comprehensiveness:* The framework is capable of offering guidance in solving a wide range of moral problems in various health care settings.
5. *Practicality:* The framework works effectively and efficiently when applied to the resolution of day-to-day ethical dilemmas in practice.

In an effort to meet the preceding criteria, the ethics decision framework proposed in this chapter was assessed by 12 graduate nursing students enrolled in a health care ethics course and by 23 nurse clinicians and administrators attending a national conference on ethical issues in nursing. The assessment took the following form: First, participants were asked to divide into small groups and appoint a recorder; second, they were asked to read the entire proposed ethics framework; third, they were asked to read a case on "Conscientious Refusal to Care for a Patient." Following reading of the case, the recorder for each group wrote down the group's assessment of the case and summarized each step of the group's decision making process based on the ethics framework. After analyzing the case, each participant was asked to evaluate the framework.

Of the 35 persons who used the framework, the vast majority of them reported that the framework helped them to make a morally justified decision regarding resolution of the ethical dilemma. Overall, however, the participants felt that the framework was too long and detailed for clinical practice. Therefore the framework was streamlined to include about half of its original items. It is this streamlined version that is presented here. Prior to this presentation, as background information, let us examine some existing ethics frameworks.

EXAMPLES OF ETHICS
DECISION FRAMEWORKS

Over the past decade several authors have offered frameworks for ethics decision making in nursing and health care (e.g., Aroskar, 1980a, 1980b; Brody, 1981; Curtin, 1982; Francoeur, 1983; Thompson & Thompson, 1985). These frameworks are discussed briefly to demonstrate examples of frameworks that nurse administrators can use separately or in conjunction with the framework formulated in this chapter.

Aroskar Framework

In the Aroskar (1980a,b) framework, an ethical dilemma is assessed in terms of three major components: (1) A *data base* that includes the actors and their histories, the setting, the proposed action, the purpose of the action, the choices and their outcomes, and the consequences of the proposed action; (2) *decision theory* that focuses on who should decide and why, what criteria should be used in making the decision, and what are the moral principles affected by the decision; and (3) *ethical theories* that focus on deontology, utilitarianism, and egoism. Underlying these three components are time considerations and the value systems of those involved in and affected by the decision.

Brody Framework

In the Brody (1981) approach to decision making, models are presented for the utilitarian ethical method and for the deontological ethical method, among others. Brody (1981, pp. 9–13) specifies the following steps in the utilitarian ethical method:

1. Perceive a moral problem exists.
2. Make a list of alternative courses of action to deal with the problem.
3. Choose one course of action as the appropriate one.
4. Frame the choice made in the form of an ethical statement (e.g., I have decided to do X, and others like me under the same circumstances ought to do X because of these consequences).
5. Determine the immediate and long-range major consequences if the proposed statement of ethics were to be accepted.
6. Compare each consequence with one's values to assess whether or not the ethical statement is consistent.

7. If one's values are inconsistent with the formulated ethical statement, reframe the ethical statement and readdress steps 5 through 7.

In contrast to the preceding utilitarian method, Brody (1981, pp. 353–354) specifies the following steps in the deontological ethical method:

1. Perceive a moral problem exists.
2. List alternative courses of action and compare these to a list of rules or principles.
3. If the comparison shows that only one alternative is consistent with the rules, that alternative is the right action.
4. If the comparison shows several alternatives are consistent with the rules, there are several right actions and one can choose among them.
5. If none of the alternatives fits the rule, or if an alternative contradicts some rules but fits others, then the decision must be made by prioritizing the importance of the rules or by appealing to a higher-level rule that may or may not resolve the conflict.

Curtin Framework

Curtin (1982, pp. 57–63), in her framework for ethical analysis, addresses some of the same components of the preceding Aroskar and Brody models, while adding others. Her analysis includes the following steps: (1) Gather, organize, and rank relevant information for the decision; (2) identify and clarify ethical components; (3) assess the rights, duties, capabilities, and authority of the decision makers; (4) determine possible courses of action and projected outcomes; (5) reconcile differing values; and (6) take action based on the preceding analysis. Curtin also recognizes that, although social expectations and legal requirements are not intrinsic to ethical decision making, they may sway the decision.

Francoeur Framework

Francoeur's (1983, pp. xvi–xvii) approach to ethics decision making consists of the following: (1) Define the problem; (2) identify pertinent moral issues and prioritize values; (3) identify alternatives and weigh them; (4) apply the decision making process; (5) choose the alternative that is most ethical and medically acceptable; and (6) carry out the decision. Throughout his book, Francoeur elaborates on each of these steps in considerable detail, including such topics as decisions in triage situations, using operational decision techniques, decision trees, and decision matrix techniques.

Thompson and Thompson Framework

Thompson and Thompson (1981, p. 13; 1985, p. 99) have formulated a bioethics decision model composed of these ten steps:

1. Review the situation to assess ethical aspects, key persons, health problems, and needed decisions.
2. Gather other information needed to clarify the situation.
3. Identify ethical issues in the situation.
4. Define professional and personal moral stances.
5. Identify moral stances of key persons involved.
6. Identify value conflicts when they exist.
7. Determine who is best able to make the decision.
8. Identify range of decisions/actions with anticipated outcome for all persons involved in the situation.
9. Decide on a course of action and implement it.
10. Evaluate results of decisions/actions.

The preceding five ethics decision frameworks have been presented not only to show diversity of approaches but also, more importantly, to show commonality of approaches. That is, all five frameworks are process oriented (i.e., they include a systematic way of thinking about the resolution of an ethical issue) and include, at a minimum, the following components: data collection and assessment, problem identification, decision and consideration of course of action, and selection of action. These four steps as well as reflection on the decision and course of action (addressed in some of the frameworks) are considered essential to ethics decision making and, therefore, are incorporated into the following ethics decision framework.

AN ETHICS DECISION FRAMEWORK

With consideration given to (1) the background information presented in Chapters 1 through 4, (2) the five criteria for a sound decision framework (adequacy, consistency, coherence, comprehensiveness, and practicality), (3) the five steps of the ethics decision process identified in the preceding paragraph, and (4) a critique of the framework by 12 graduate nursing students and 23 nurse clinicians and administrators, the refined ethics framework is now presented. The major goal of the framework is to assist nurse administrators to assess an ethical dilemma in a systematic manner, arriving at a morally justified decision based on accurate facts, relevant knowledge, and sound reasoning. The framework should help nurse administrators become clearer on the nature of ethical dilemmas and on courses of action that are morally justifiable. The framework, however, has limits. It does not automatically lead to *a* morally right action; it may lead to *more than one* morally right action. In addition, the framework may lead to *morally wrong* actions if the decision makers are faulty in their moral reasoning. With these caveats in mind, we will now examine the five steps of the framework.

Data Collection and Assessment

Data collection and assessment of those data are integral and ongoing parts of the decision making process for resolution of an ethical dilemma in nursing. Categories of data, with examples of assessment questions, include the following.

I. DATA COLLECTION AND ASSESSMENT OF DATA

A. Situational Considerations
   1. What situational factors contribute to the ethical dilemma or issue?
   2. How do these situational factors contribute to the ethical dilemma or issue?
B. Health Team Considerations
   1. What persons are most involved in the situation?
   2. What are the relevant backgrounds (e.g., educational level, value orientations) of the persons most involved?
   3. What persons are most affected by the outcome of the decision?
C. Organizational Considerations
   1. What is the nature and mission of the organization?
   2. What are the organization's values, policies, and procedures relevant to the situation?

In review, the data collection and assessment include, but are not limited to, one or more of the preceding categories in interaction with one another. Each consideration is addressed briefly regarding how it affects ethics decision making.

In situational considerations, one must determine whether it reflects an ethical dilemma or another type of dilemma. For example, a decision about whether a new wing of a hospital should be painted a pastel blue or green may present an aesthetic dilemma, but it does not normally present an ethical dilemma. Whether a patient should be assisted to dress now or an hour from now may pose an organizational dilemma but does not normally pose an ethical dilemma. On the other hand, whether health care providers should intervene in the planned suicide of a seemingly rational patient does pose an ethical dilemma.

Regarding health team considerations, one must determine what persons will be affected by the decision and how the decision will affect their lives. Knowing background information about the persons involved in, or affected by, the decision will give insight into their way of thinking about the dilemma. As discussed in Chapter 4, educational level, stages of moral development, and values ascribed to, all contribute to how a person thinks and makes decisions about ethical dilemmas.

With organizational considerations, one must remember that policies and procedures frequently affect how ethical dilemmas get resolved. As such, these organizational policies and procedures may place constraints on nurses. These constraints have been discussed by Davis and Aroskar (1983, p. 49), who view the problem as follows: "The overriding ethical issue for nurses, especially those working in hospitals, can best be described as one of multiple obligations coupled with the question of authority." These multiple obligations and authority conflicts raise the question of what is the nurse's ethical obligation, and how far does the nurse go to fulfill this obligation?

As noted in Chapter 4, Swider, McElmurry, and Yarling (1985) found that baccalaureate nursing students' decisions in solving an ethical dilemma were bureaucracy-centered 60 percent of the time, physician-centered 19 percent of the time, patient-centered 9 percent of the time, and other-centered 12 percent of the time. When only first decisions were assessed, however, 89 percent were bureaucracy-centered. The bureaucracy appears to be an important determiner of the type of decisions that will emerge in resolving ethical dilemmas in institutional settings. Therefore, it is important that nurse administrators ensure that nursing policies and procedures are ethical. Furthermore, it is important that nurse administrators recognize that policies and procedures do *not* represent the highest levels of moral justification. These highest levels—ethical theories and principles—were discussed in Chapters 2 and 3.

Problem Identification

Adequate resolution of dilemmas cannot occur without a clear understanding of the nature of the problem. Examples of questions that one can ask to identify and clarify a problem related to ethics include the following.

II. PROBLEM IDENTIFICATION

A. Ethical Considerations
    1. What are ethical considerations related to the problem?
    2. Which of these ethical considerations take priority?
B. Nonethical Considerations
    1. What are nonethical considerations related to the problem (e.g., medical, legal, or factual considerations)?
    2. How do the nonethical considerations relate to the ethical considerations?

As outlined above, problem identification includes obtaining clarity on both the ethical and nonethical considerations relevant to the problem, as well as the interrelationship between the two. Regarding the ethical considerations relevant to the problem, it is important to analyze the precise ethical issues involved. Some situations are complex; therefore, several ethical issues may be involved. For example, the primary ethical issue may be whether or not to tell the truth; however, this issue often generates other simultaneous ethical issues related to conflicts of obligations and values. Therefore, it is necessary to first identify all the relevant ethical issues. Once these issues are identified, they can then be prioritized in terms of primary and secondary issues.

Thompson and Thompson (1985) have categorized ethical issues as follows.

Examples of Ethical Issues[1]

Issues of Principle:

1. Autonomy, self-determination of patients and professionals.
2. Do good, do no harm (beneficence, nonmaleficence).
3. Justice, fairness (allocation of resources).
4. Truth-telling (veracity).
5. Informed consent.
6. Quality of life/sanctity of life.
7. The Golden Rule.

Issues of Ethical Rights:

1. Right to privacy (confidentiality).
2. Right to decide what happens to oneself/one's body (self-determination).
3. Right to health care (currently debatable; some say equal access only, others say not a right at all).
4. Right to information (informed consent, access to records).
5. Right to choose whom you care for (frequently limited to physicians in nonemergency situations).
6. Right to live, right to die.
7. Rights of children.

Issues of Ethical Duties/Obligations:

1. Respect persons.
2. Be accountable for decisions/actions.
3. Maintain competence (professionals).
4. Exercise informed judgment in professional practice.
5. Implement and improve standards of profession.
6. Participate in activities contributing to profession's knowledge base.
7. Safeguard clients from incompetent, unethical, or illegal practice of any person.
8. Promote efforts to meet health needs of public.
9. Participate in the formulation of public policy.

---

[1]**From:** Thompson, J. E., & Thompson, H. O. (1985). *Bioethical decision making for nurses* (pp. 121–122). Norwalk, CT: Appleton–Century–Crofts.

Issues of Ethical Loyalty:

1. Professional–patient relationship (covenant fidelity, contract, seller of services).
2. Accountability to whom as employee.
3. Professional–professional relationships.
4. Professional–patient family relationship.
5. Who decides.

Issues of Concern in Life Cycle:

1. Contraception and sterilization.
2. Genetic engineering and embryo transfer.
3. Abortion (When does life begin?).
4. Infanticide.
5. Adolescent sexuality.
6. Allocation of scarce resources.
7. Lifestyle.
8. Euthanasia.

In our professional role, our first priority is the patient. As stated in the American Nurses' Association's *Code for Nurses* (1985, p. 6), "The nurse's primary commitment is to the health, welfare, and safety of the client." Therefore resolution of ethical issues affecting the client usually takes precedence over ethical issues affecting others. In the case where a decision needs to be made about whether or not the patient should be told the truth, it is obvious the nurse cannot act and the patient cannot benefit from this action until the decision is made. The making of the decision may involve resolution of professionals' conflicting obligations and values. This resolution is important because usually the patient cannot benefit from the action until the resolution occurs. Long-standing conflicts among professionals, however, regarding obligations and values *not* related to the resolution of the immediate ethical dilemma should not cloud the decision making process. Resolution of these other dilemmas are important but may not be the top priority.

Regarding nonethical considerations, it is important to remember that the analysis and resolution of ethical dilemmas are often affected by, for example, factual considerations. Ethical theories and principles carry us so far; although they provide a useful organizing framework and helpful moral content with which to structure a dilemma, they lack the specific data needed to give substance to the resolution of the dilemma.

Consideration of Possible Actions

Once the ethical problem is identified, viable actions must be considered before a decision is reached. Viable actions include the following:

1. Actions that can be morally justified.
2. Actions relevant to the resolution of the dilemma.
3. Actions that are implementable.

Within these boundaries, a utilitarian and a deontological approach to the consideration of actions are presented.

III. CONSIDERATION OF POSSIBLE ACTIONS

A. Utilitarian Thinking
   1. How is the principle of utility being defined (e.g., happiness, pleasure, health, etc)?
   2. What are viable actions?
   3. What are predicted consequences of the actions for persons affected by the decision?
   4. From the predicted consequences, what is the intrinsic value and disvalue for each viable consequence?
   5. What possible action(s) produce the best consequences overall for happiness, pleasure, health, etc and the least unhappiness, disvalue, displeasure, etc for persons affected, or most affected, by the decision?
B. Deontological Thinking
   1. What ethical rules and principles are in conflict?[2]
   2. What duties emerge from these ethical rules and principles?
   3. Which of these duties are in conflict with equal or stronger duties?
   4. If a conflict exists, which duties derived from moral rules and principles produce the greatest balance of rightness over wrongness?

---

[2]**Note:** A rule utilitarian would also raise questions about ethical rules and principles, but would assess the rules in terms of consequences instead of duties.

Regarding utilitarian thinking, the following points discussed in Chapter 2 should be remembered:

- Utilitarianism is a moral theory whose proponents endorse the premise that no acts are right or wrong except by reference to the consequences produced by the acts.
- Desired consequences maximize intrinsic values for all persons affected by the act; undesirable consequences diminish intrinsic values for all persons affected by the act.
- The right act (that is, the one that we are morally obligated to follow) is the one whose consequences produce the most net pleasure minus pain for all persons affected by, or most affected by, the act.

Francoeur (1983), in adapting the utilitarian decision making model developed by Brody (1981), offers the flow chart seen in Figure 5–1 for consequence-oriented ethics decision making.

Regarding deontologogical thinking, the following points discussed in Chapter 2 should be remembered:

- Deontology is a moral theory whose proponents endorse the premise that features of acts other than, or in addition to, their consequences determine the rightness or wrongness of an act.
- Features of acts other than consequences that determine an act's rightness or wrongness include duties, rights, virtues, and motives.
- The right act (that is, the one that we are morally obligated to follow) is the one required by duty.
- When equally stringent duties conflict, the right act is the one that produces the greatest balance of rightness over wrongness.

Francoeur (1983), in adapting the deontological decision making model developed by Brody (1981), offers the flow chart seen in Figure 5–2 for duty-oriented ethics decision making.

In summary, morally justifiable actions can be arrived at by using either utilitarian or deontological thinking. Theoretically one cannot be both; however, in reality persons sometimes use a mixture of the two, or use utilitarian thinking in one situation and deontological thinking in another situation. For example, utilitarian thinking is often used in resolving ethical dilemmas regarding allocation of scarce resources; deontological thinking is often used in resolving ethical dilemmas involving informed consent. In addition, it is important to remember the purpose of ethical theory: to provide a broad orientation to a set of

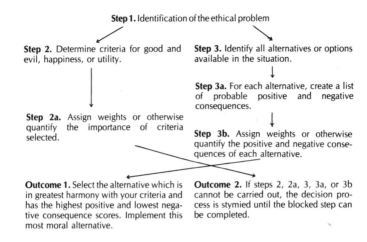

Figure 5–1 A consequence-oriented process for ethics decision making.
From: Francoeur, R. T. (1983). *Biomedical ethics: A guide to decision making* (p. 10). New York: Wiley. Reprinted with permission of John Wiley & Sons, Inc. Adapted from the following original source: Brody, H. (1981). *Ethical decisions in medicine* (2nd ed.). Boston: Little, Brown.

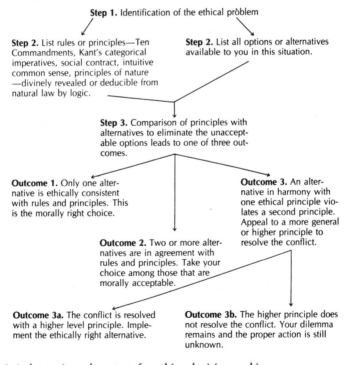

Figure 5–2 A duty-oriented process for ethics decision making.
From: Francoeur, R. T. (1983). *Biomedical ethics: A guide to decision making* (p.9). New York: Wiley. Reprinted with permission of John Wiley & Sons, Inc. Adapted from the following original source: Brody, H. (1981). *Ethical decisions in medicine* (2nd ed.). Boston: Little, Brown.

beliefs that facilitate study of the moral life. Ethical theory also represents the highest level of moral justification. Nevertheless, despite this strength, it does not provide answers; only the decision makers themselves can determine morally justified responses to ethical dilemmas.

Decision and Selection of Course of Action

Once data have been collected and assessed, the ethical problem identified, and potential actions considered, it is time to make a decision. Jameton (1984) offers a sobering thought on this part of the decision making process:

> Those who turn to ethics in the hope of finding a secure and definite action are bound to be disappointed. There is no way to escape the final responsibility of saying, "This is my choice." (p. 68)

To help facilitate making a choice, the following questions are suggested.

IV. DECISION AND SELECTION OF COURSE OF ACTION

A. Contribution of Internal/Group Factors
   1. For whom is the decision being made?
   2. Who should decide?
   3. What biases/values of persons involved in the situation affect the decision?
B. Contribution of External Factors
   1. What institutional factors are affecting the decision and selected course of action?
   2. What legal factors are affecting the decision and selected course of action?
   3. What social factors are affecting the decision and selected course of action?
C. Quality of Decision and Course of Action
   1. What decision is being made?
   2. What course of action to implement the decision is being made?
   3. In light of the preceding factors, is the decision being made and the course of action to be taken ones that can still be morally justified?

4. If not, how can the decision being made and the course of action to be taken be altered so that they are morally justified?
5. Is the selected course of action based on the decision implementable?

Regarding internal/group factors, one must remember that decision making is a complex process and that people do not make decisions in the way predicted by mathematical models. There is always the issue of human biases and values that affect both the decision making process and the decision. If nurse administrators and others involved in the decision recognize their biases and values, a less emotional and more rational decision may be made.

When several persons are involved in a decision, value conflicts can occur. To help resolve such conflicts, persons should reflect upon the assessment questions and guidelines discussed in the values conflict section of Chapter 4. In addition, Curtin (1982) offers some guidance for conflicting opinions:

> If there are conflicting conclusions among various participants in a shared decision, one may have to defer to the person who is affected most directly by the decision. Although people never should undertake an action they sincerely believe to be wrong (for that is the definition of immorality), they should weigh all factors carefully before withdrawing or blocking decision making. There are times when both of these activities are appropriate, but sometimes acquiescing to the will of the majority is the best course of action. Where is the greater good or the lesser harm? Is the problem better served by one's withdrawal or participation? Is the situation best handled by submission to the authority of the group? Sometimes a person may have to stand alone. On no account should dissenters be forced to comply against their will or be denigrated in any way. Even when the group members cannot agree with a dissenter, they can understand how and why the person dissents. No matter what decision must be made, it cannot assume more importance than the people making it, lest people be sacrificed for the principles designed to protect them. Even if they cannot agree with a group's decision, dissenters can come to understand how and why the group reached a particular decision. (p. 63). (Reprinted with permission)

Regarding external factors, it is important to identify when and how legal, institutional, and social ramifications impinge upon and either positively or negatively affect ethical decisions. If one believes in the mark of the moral discussed in Chapter 1 that "morality overrides other human values," then care must be taken that extrinsic factors do not sway decisions so that their morality is compromised.

Once a morally justified decision is made, it must be implemented. As previously noted, no decision should be made that cannot be implemented in practice; an unimplemented decision does not resolve an ethical dilemma. Impediments to such implementation could be insufficient funds or personnel to carry out the decision. Thus a practical orientation, in addition to a theoretical one, is important in formulating a morally justified *and* implementable action to resolve an ethical dilemma.

Reflection on Decision and Course of Action

Once the decision is implemented, the course of action taken to implement the decision should be assessed to determine whether the intended action occurred in the manner intended and whether the intended action accomplished its purpose. If the intended action accomplished its purpose in the manner intended, resolution of the ethical dilemma will presumably have occurred. One of the following problems, however, could occur:

1. The action was *not* implemented as intended.
2. The action was implemented as intended, but an *un*intended result occurred.

In either case the intended purpose could be compromised or not achieved. Under these circumstances, resolution of the ethical dilemma most likely will *not* have occurred, and new problem solving strategies must be devised.

To facilitate assessment of the ethics decision and course of action, the following questions are suggested.

V. REFLECTION ON DECISION AND COURSE OF ACTION

A. Reflection on Decision
   1. Was the decision that was made the one that was actually acted upon? If not, why not?

2. Did the decision that was made accomplish its intended purpose? If not, why not?
3. In retrospect, do you believe the decision that was made was morally good or right? Why? Why not?

B. Reflection on Course of Action
1. Was the selected course of action carried out in the manner intended? If not, why not?
2. Did the selected course of action accomplish its intended purpose? If not, why not?
3. In retrospect, do you believe the course of action taken was morally good or right? Why? Why not?

The preceding five-step ethics decision framework provides nurse administrators with one approach to the analysis, potential resolution, and evaluation of ethical dilemmas. The framework provides a process by which moral reasoning and moral justification can be facilitated.

Summary. In this chapter, five criteria for validation of an ethics decision framework are discussed: (1) adequacy, (2) consistency, (3) coherence, (4) comprehensiveness, and (5) practicality. In addition, several ethics decision frameworks are reviewed to determine important components. These components are: (1) data collection and assessment, (2) problem identification, (3) consideration of actions, (4) decision and selection of course of action, and (5) reflection on decision and course of action. These components serve as the organizing framework for the ethics decision framework developed herein. The framework was validated by both graduate nursing students and professional nurses. In Chapters 6 through 8 the framework is applied to ethical dilemmas in nursing administration.

REFERENCES

American Nurses' Association. (1985). *Code for nurses with interpretive statements.* Kansas City, MO: Author.

Aroskar, M. A. (1980a). Anatomy of an ethical dilemma: The theory. *American Journal of Nursing, 80,* 658–660.

Aroskar, M. A. (1980b). Anatomy of an ethical dilemma: The practice. *American Journal of Nursing, 80,* 661–663.

Brody, H. (1981). *Ethical decisions in medicine* (2nd ed.). Boston: Little, Brown.

Curtin, L. (1982). No rush to judgment. In L. Curtin & M. J. Flaherty, *Nursing ethics: Theories and pragmatics* (pp. 57–63). Bowie, MD: Brady.

Davis, A. J., & Aroskar, M. A. (1983). *Ethical dilemmas and nursing practice* (2nd ed.). Norwalk, CT: Appleton–Century–Crofts.

Francoeur, R. T. (1983). *Biomedical ethics: A guide to decision making.* New York: Wiley.

Jameton, A. (1984). *Nursing practice: The ethical issues.* Englewood Cliffs, NJ: Prentice-Hall.

Swider, S. M., McElmurry, B. J., & Yarling, R. R. (1985). Ethical decision making in a bureaucratic context by senior nursing students. *Nursing Research, 34,* 108–112.

Thompson, J. B., & Thompson, H. O. (1981). *Ethics in nursing.* New York: MacMillian.

Thompson, J. E., & Thompson, H. O. (1985). *Bioethical decision making for nurses.* Norwalk, CT: Appleton–Century–Crofts.

Principle of Autonomy Versus Principle of Beneficence: Case Analyses

Mary Cipriano Silva
and Helen M. Jenkins

Man will ever stand in
need of man.
                    Theocritus

In Chapters 1 through 5, basic content related to ethics is discussed. That content will be applied to actual case situations faced by an Assistant Director for Home Health Services and a former Division Chief Nurse at a large psychiatric hospital. The cases, which focus on a conflict between the ethical principle of autonomy and the ethical principle of beneficence, will be reflected upon by applying the ethics decision framework presented in Chapter 5. This framework is summarized as follows:

Ethics Decision Framework

I. Data Collection and Assessment
   A. Situational Considerations
   B. Health Team Considerations
   C. Organizational Considerations
II. Problem Identification
   A. Ethical Considerations
   B. Nonethical Considerations
III. Consideration of Possible Actions
   A. Utilitarian Thinking
   B. Deontological Thinking
IV. Decision and Selection of Course of Action
   A. Contribution of Internal/Group Factors

  B. Contribution of External Factors
  C. Quality of Decision and Course of Action
V. Reflection on Decision and Course of Action
  A. Reflection on Decision
  B. Reflection on Course of Action

In using the framework, one must remember that the categories are basic but not exhaustive. In addition, because the framework is used as a heuristic device, some content is repeated to emphasize important points. With practice, however, it is assumed that repetition will not be needed and the steps of the framework will be integrated into one's practice with ease and efficiency.

| CASE STUDY 1 |

The Terminally Ill Suicidal Patient[1]

For three years, Mr J had cancer of the testes with metastasis to the bladder, rectum, perineum, and lungs. He had a colostomy, suprapubic catheter, and perineal wounds. Toward the end of his life, he was bedridden, in great pain, and had pain-relieving medication at his bedside that could be taken as needed but was insufficient to relieve the pain. He was 65 years old.

Mr J was intelligent and had a broad range of federal government experience. Despite his terminal illness, he was rational and tried to maintain as normal a life as possible. He clearly stated to his wife and physician that he wanted no heroics taken to save his life and had written a living will. In addition, he had told them that he wanted to die if the pain and lack of independence became overwhelming. He also had discussed the possibility of suicide with his wife, who was supportive of suicide if this was what he wanted.

Mrs J was a physician who worked during the week but took care of her husband on weekends. Although the duration of her husband's illness had left Mrs J fatigued and depressed, she maintained frequent communication with Mr J's doctor. Their major goal was to control Mr J's pain. Mr and Mrs J had no children.

During the last year of his life, Mr and Mrs J had contracted for patient care services from the Visiting Nurse Association (VNA). The patient care services

---

[1]**Case Submitted by: Ruby Van Croft, RN, MS,** Director for Special Programs, Visiting Nurse Association, Washington, D.C.

included a registered nurse who visited Mr J twice a day as needed, Mondays through Fridays. The registered nurse provided Mr J with perineal wound care, colostomy care, and also monitored his pain.

In addition to the VNA services, Mr and Mrs J contracted for care from a home health aide. On one visit, the home health aide told the VNA nurse that she had overheard Mr J dictate a note to his wife about his plans to commit suicide. The nurse was upset by this information and felt a conflict between her belief that suicide was wrong and her belief that terminally ill, suffering patients should be able to choose their own time and way to die. When she returned to the office, the nurse shared the information about Mr J's planned suicide with her supervisor. The supervisor in turn shared the information with the Assistant Director for Home Health Services at the VNA.

The Assistant Director advised the nurse to notify Mr J's physician and his wife of the situation. At the time the VNA had no policies to cover the terminally ill suicidal patient, and the Assistant Director consulted the agency lawyer to learn about the agency's legal responsibility. Since Mr J's planned death was *not* considered natural, the lawyer advised the Assistant Director that an ambulance should be called and the patient taken to the hospital in the event of a suicide attempt.

The next day when the nurse visited Mr J, she found him unresponsive and ascertained that he had taken an overdose of his pain-relieving medication. She was unable to do anything for him except call an ambulance. When Mrs J was notified, she requested that the nurse cancel the ambulance and allow her husband to die in peace. Based on the recently obtained legal advice, however, the nurse felt she could not cancel the ambulance. The patient was taken to the hospital where he died without gaining consciousness.

DATA COLLECTION AND ASSESSMENT

I. Data Collection and Assessment
  A. Situational Considerations
    1. What situational factors contribute to the ethical dilemma or issue?
    2. How do these situational factors contribute to the ethical dilemma or issue?
  B. Health Team Considerations
    1. What persons are most involved in the situation?
    2. What are the relevant backgrounds (e.g., educational level, value orientations) of the persons most involved?

3. What persons are most affected by the outcome of the decision?
C. Organizational Considerations
1. What is the nature and mission of the organization?
2. What are the organization's values, policies, and procedures
relevant to the situation?

Situational Considerations

The situational factors contributing to the ethical dilemma, and their
method of contribution, are as follows:

1. *Mr J was suicidal.* The underlying ethical issue is whether suicide
is ever morally justified and, if so, under what conditions. In
particular, does terminal illness involving loss of dignity and
great suffering without relief of pain constitute a morally justifiable reason for suicide?
2. *Mrs J was aware that her husband was suicidal.* Because Mrs J was
both aware and supportive of her husband's contemplated suicide, the following ethical issue must be raised: Is being supportive of suicide (either actively or passively) ever morally justified
and, if so, under what conditions? In particular, does terminal
illness involving loss of dignity and great suffering without relief of pain constitute a morally justifiable reason for a family
member to encourage or support another family member in
committing suicide?
3. *Mr J was receiving contracted-for care.* The aide, nurse, and Assistant Director would not have been involved in this ethical
dilemma if the family had not contracted to receive care from a
home health aide and from the VNA. Since a major responsibility of health providers in caring for terminally ill patients is to
provide comfort to the dying and their families but not to contribute deliberately to the patient's death, did the patient and
his wife violate the contract (i.e., break a promise)? On the other
hand, did the home health aide violate the patient's right to
privacy by listening, albeit by chance, to his dictated suicide
message?
4. *Mr J had access to pain-relieving medication in sufficient dosage to
commit suicide.* Mr J could not have committed suicide by pain-
relieving medications if these had not been available to him.
What is the moral obligation of the physician in prescribing

pain-relieving medications to terminally ill and potentially suicidal patients? Under these latter circumstances, what is the moral obligation, if any, of a nurse to restrict the patient from having full access to these drugs? What is the moral obligation of the patient to take these medications only in the amount and for the reasons prescribed?

Health Team Considerations

Persons most involved in the situation were Mr J, his wife, the lawyer, and the Assistant Director of the VNA, who made the final nursing decision in the situation. Other persons involved included the visiting nurse, physician, and aide.

Relevant information for persons most involved include:

1. *Mr J*—At age 62 Mr J had a total excision of his perineal area for cancer of the testes, with metastasis to his bladder, rectum, perineum, and lungs. In addition, he had a colostomy, suprapubic catheter, and perineal wounds. By age 65 he was bedridden and in great pain. Several pain-relieving medications, including talwin and morphine, had been ordered for him at various times by his physician, but the medication was inadequate to control his pain. Mr J was an intelligent and independent man who maintained his independence as long as possible. He did not want heroic measures taken to preserve his life, however, and had written a living will stating so. His thinking was considered rational by those who cared for him. His religious affiliation was unknown.

2. *Mrs J*—Mrs J was a physician who took care of her husband on weekends. To care for Mr J during the week, she hired a home health aide and also contracted for nursing care from the VNA. She was in frequent communication with Mr J's physician to try to control his pain. She was aware of the possibility of Mr J's suicide and was supportive of it. She wanted her husband to die in peace.

3. *The lawyer*—The lawyer was an important member of the health team in this situation because he offered advice about the course of action to be taken. That is, he advised that in the event of a suicide attempt, an ambulance should be called, and Mr J should be taken to the hospital.

4. *The Assistant Director*—The Assistant Director found this case difficult for several reasons. First, the VNA had no policy that dealt with terminally ill suicidal patients. Second, she felt torn

between honoring the request of the patient and his wife regarding the suicide and her own personal feelings that suicide was wrong. Third, she had no prior experience with this type of situation and had little time for reflection as immediate action was needed. Fourth, she knew first hand how much suffering was involved in watching a loved one die from terminal cancer as she had experienced the situation in her own family.

The person most affected by the outcome of the decision was Mr J, whose life was at stake. His wife was also profoundly affected by the decision as Mr J's death would leave her a widow. The lawyer and the Assistant Director were affected by the decision insofar as their personal integrity and that of their agency were at stake.

Organizational Considerations

The goal of the District of Columbia's Visiting Nurse Association is to provide care in the patient's home and to maintain the patient's maximum level of independence. When persons are dying, the goal is to help them die in their own homes in comfort but without actively assisting them to die. If dying patients have requested a natural death, they are permitted to die normally without heroics or an ambulance being called, although the coroner must be notified. As previously noted, at the time of this case there was no agency policy in the event of death by suicide.

PROBLEM IDENTIFICATION

II. Problem Identification
  A. Ethical Considerations
     1. What are ethical considerations related to the case?
     2. Which of these ethical considerations take priority?
  B. Nonethical Considerations
     1. What are nonethical considerations related to the case (e.g., medical, legal, or factual considerations)?
     2. How do the nonethical considerations relate to the ethical considerations?

Ethical Considerations

Major ethical considerations in the case are as follows:

1. *In regard to Mr J*—Is it permissible for Mr J to take his own life? If yes, what means are morally acceptable?
2. *In regard to Mrs J*—Should Mrs J encourage or support Mr J in taking his own life?
3. *In regard to the Assistant Director*—Should the Assistant Director, in the absence of agency policy, encourage the nurse to respect the patient's autonomous wish to commit suicide or encourage the nurse to prevent the suicide?

Nonethical Considerations

The major nonethical considerations in this case were legal ones. The Assistant Director contacted an agency lawyer because of the lack of agency policy regarding suicidal patients. The lawyer stated that, in the eyes of the law, suicides or attempted suicides were viewed differently from natural deaths. That is, in suicides or attempted suicides an ambulance should be called and the patient taken to the hospital; in natural deaths these measures were unnecessary.

CONSIDERATION OF POSSIBLE ACTIONS: UTILITARIAN THINKING

III. Consideration of Possible Actions
   A. Utilitarian Thinking
   1. How is the principle of utility being defined in this case (e.g., happiness, pleasure, health, etc)?
   2. What are viable actions in the case?
   3. What are predicted consequences of the actions for persons affected by the decision?
   4. From the predicted consequences, what is the intrinsic value and disvalue for each viable consequence?
   5. What possible action(s) produce the best consequences overall for happiness, pleasure, health, etc and the least unhappiness, disvalue, displeasure, etc for persons affected, or most affected, by the decision?

Definition of the Principle of Utility

To review, the principle of utility according to Mill (1861/1979, p. 7) "holds that actions are right in proportion as they tend to promote happiness; wrong as they tend to produce the reverse of happiness." In this case the principle of utility is being applied differently. For Mr J, utility is primarily freedom from the physical pain of terminal cancer and the psychological pain of loss of dignity. For Mrs J, utility is not only a desire to see Mr J's physical and psychological pain alleviated but also a desire to diminish her own pain in seeing a loved one suffer. The Assistant Director's understanding of utility, however, is most closely associated with agency policy related to maintenance of health and life.

As noted in Chapter 2, utility can be conceived entirely in terms of happiness or pleasure (or freedom from unhappiness or pain) or in terms of other intrinsic values such as knowledge, love, beauty, or health. Therefore, as shown in this case, conflict may occur at the first step of utilitarian thinking (i.e., definition of and agreement on the utility at stake): Persons most involved in or affected by a given situation may not agree on what counts as utility.

Viable Actions

Viable actions to consider in this case include the following:

1. Allow Mr J to take his own life.
2. Allow Mrs J to support her husband in taking his own life.
3. Prevent Mr J from taking his own life.

The principle of utility requires that one assess the consequences of possible actions to determine their impact on the welfare of all persons affected by the action. In terms of utilitarian thinking, the argument for suicide often goes as follows: If the value of relief from pain by taking one's own life is greater than the value to society of one's continued existence, then suicide is justifiable and may even be admirable if directed at benefit to others. For further discussions of the moral reasons for and against suicide, see Brandt (1986, pp. 337–343) and Veatch and Fry (1987, pp. 169–173).

Predicted Consequences

For the persons most affected by the decision, predicted consequences are as follows:

	Suicide allowed	Suicide prevented
1. *For Mr J*	• loss of his life • anticipated freedom from pain	• continued pain and loss of dignity • continued pain of seeing his wife suffer • continued depletion of finances
2. *For Mrs J*	• relief from the pain of seeing a loved one suffer • widowhood and concomitant loss and grief - • possible guilt over supporting husband in suicide	• mental anguish at seeing a loved one suffer • helplessness
3. *For Assistant Director of Nursing*	• violation of own conscience • violation of anticipated agency policy • violation of law	• pain of seeing a patient suffer • pain of not honoring family request for suicide • maintenance of personal and professional integrity

Intrinsic Value/Disvalue of Consequences

The primary intrinsic value for Mr J is freedom from pain. The primary intrinsic value for Mrs J is to decrease her husband's pain and, in so doing, to express the intrinsic value of love. The primary intrinsic value for the Assistant Director is maintenance of life.

Outcomes of Actions Regarding Happiness/Unhappiness

For Mr and Mrs J the greatest happiness would occur if he took his own life because only this could bring immediate relief from his pain and suffering. For the Assistant Director the greatest happiness would occur if Mr J died naturally rather than through suicide; thereby the health professionals' role to maintain life or to assist in a peaceful *natural* death would not be compromised.

CONSIDERATION OF POSSIBLE ACTIONS: DEONTOLOGICAL THINKING

III. Consideration of Possible Actions, continued
  B. Deontological Thinking
    1. What ethical rules and principles are in conflict?[2]
    2. What duties emerge from these ethical rules and principles?
    3. Which of these duties are in conflict with equal or stronger duties?
    4. If a conflict exists, which duties derived from moral rules and principles produce the greatest balance of rightness over wrongness?

Ethical Rules and Principles in Conflict

Major ethical rules and/or principles in conflict in this case are as follows:

1. *In regard to Mr J*—The principle of autonomy (i.e., Mr J's autonomous desire to commit suicide) is in conflict with the principle of sanctity of human life and that aspect of the principle of beneficence that focuses on the noninfliction of harm.

2. *In regard to Mrs J*—The principle of respect for autonomy (i.e., Mrs J's desire to support her husband's suicide) is in conflict with the principle of sanctity of human life and that aspect of the principle of beneficence that focuses on the noninfliction of harm.

3. *In regard to the Assistant Director*—The principle of respect for autonomy (i.e., respecting Mr J's wishes) is in conflict with the principle of sanctity of human life and those aspects of the principle of beneficence that focus on the noninfliction of harm and the prevention of harm. In addition, the principle of respect for autonomy is in conflict with the rule of fidelity to uphold morally justifiable agency policy regarding care of patients.

---

[2]**Note:** A rule utilitarian would also raise questions about ethical rules and principles but would assess the rules in terms of consequences instead of duties.

Duties Emerging from Rules and Principles

In this case, prima facie duties emerging from the various principles are as follows:

1. From the principle of autonomy arises the duty to act in accord with one's autonomous choices.
2. From the principle of respect for autonomy arises the duty not to interfere in the autonomous choice of others.
3. From the principle of sanctity of life arises the duty to value and preserve human life.
4. From the principle of beneficence arise the duties not to inflict harm and/or to prevent harm.
5. From the rule of fidelity arises the duty to keep promises.

Duties in Conflict

In this case, Mr and Mrs J seemingly resolved any conflicts of ethical principles or duties they had experienced regarding suicide. The VNA staff nurse, her supervisor, and the Assistant Director, however, experienced the following conflict of prima facie duties:

A conflict between the duty of allowing a terminally ill, suffering, but rational patient to choose his own time and way to die (respect for autonomy) and the duty to value and preserve human life through the noninfliction or prevention of harm.

Since the staff nurse turned to her supervisor for guidance and the supervisor turned to the Assistant Director, the primary burden of making a morally justifiable decision rested with the Assistant Director.

Greatest Balance of Rightness Over Wrongness

For Mr J the moral duty to act in accord with his autonomous choice (i.e., suicide) and for Mrs J the moral duty to respect this choice produced more rightness than the continued prolongation of Mr J's life. For the Assistant Director the moral duties to value and preserve human life and to prevent harm to this life took precedence over (and produced more rightness) than the duty to act in accord with the patient's autonomous choice. The Assistant Director's position can be supported in terms of justified paternalism if one believes the harm prevented in the case (i.e., loss of Mr J's life) outweighed the assault on his autonomy *or* if one believes that Mr J's serious illness and unrelenting pain limited his ability to make an autonomous choice.

DECISION AND SELECTION OF COURSE
OF ACTION

IV. Decision and Selection of Course of Action
    A. Contribution of Internal/Group Factors
        1. For whom is the decision being made?
        2. Who should decide?
        3. What biases/values of persons involved in the situation affect the decision?
    B. Contribution of External Factors
        1. What institutional factors are affecting the decision and selected course of action?
        2. What legal factors are affecting the decision and selected course of action?
        3. What social factors are affecting the decision and selected course of action?
    C. Quality of Decision and Course of Action
        1. What decision is being made?
        2. What course of action to implement the decision is being made?
        3. In light of the preceding factors, is the decision being made and the course of action to be taken ones that can still be morally justified?
        4. If not, how can the decision being made and the course of action to be taken be altered so that they are morally justifiable?
        5. Is the selected course of action based on the decision implementable?

Contribution of Internal/Group Factors

As discussed in Chapter 4, decision making involves human judgment and choice. These processes are affected by internal and personal factors such as values and educational level. In this case Mr J is the focus of the decision making process, but this focus is somewhat different for Mr and Mrs J than it is for the Assistant Director. For Mr and Mrs J the decision of Mr J to commit suicide is primarily a personal matter (value) mutually agreed upon by husband and wife in order to stop Mr J's pain. Since Mr and Mrs J have no children, the normal adverse effects of a parental suicide are irrelevant in *this* case, although there are those who would argue that the suicide of any human being diminishes all human beings. The Assistant Director, however, by virtue of her role, must be concerned with a decision that not only affects Mr J but all similar patients to whom the agency must render care. This concern about similar patients in relevantly similar situations is in keeping with the criterion of morality that focuses on universalizability (Beauchamp, 1982, p. 13). (*See* Chapter 1.)

Who should decide is difficult to answer. Remember that nursing became involved in this case because the home health aide hired by Mr and Mrs J inadvertently overheard Mr J dictate a suicide note to his wife. Otherwise Mr J would have committed suicide without interference from health professionals. The aide and consequently the nurse, supervisor, and Assistant Director, however, *did* hear about the planned suicide. This knowledge complicated the situation because these persons represented agencies that had entered into contractual arrangements with Mr and Mrs J to provide nursing care to Mr J. This care operated on two levels—explicit and implicit. Explicit care included such activities as the colostomy care and perineal wound care. Implicit care included not taking any actions *or* preventing any actions that, without producing benefits, could harm Mr J. Since Mr J's intent was to actively and seriously harm himself and cause his death, his care and contract with the agencies would be compromised. Therefore the agencies also had a legitimate decision making claim.

The underlying values in this case represent the struggle between the principles of respect for autonomy and for the sanctity of human life. Mr J, intelligent and rational, made a decision for autonomous suicide. He decided that death was preferable to prolonged suffering without relief. Mr J's situation represents perhaps the strongest case for autonomous suicide. He was rational and ready to die; his illness was terminal and hard to manage; his pain was uncontrollable; and his suffering was severe and prolonged.

On the other hand the Assistant Director, although sympathetic to Mr J's wishes and condition, had strong personal and religious values against the taking of one's own life. In addition she felt a violation of her professional obligation to Mr J if she allowed him to commit suicide, albeit autonomously.

Contribution of External Factors

In this case legal considerations were the dominant external factor. As previously noted, the lawyer advised that in the event of Mr J's attempted suicide, an ambulance should be called and the patient taken to the hospital. This advice was the most powerful factor affecting the Assistant Director's mode of operating as it was this information that was communicated to the VNA nurse caring for Mr J.

Quality of Decision and Course of Action

The decision was made to save Mr J's life; the decision was acted upon by taking him to a hospital by ambulance. Although this course of action was implementable, it was also controversial, especially since Mrs J did not want her husband taken to the hospital. Proponents of weak paternalism could morally justify the preceding decision by stating their conviction that the good (preservation of life) was greater than the harm (death by one's own hand) and that Mr J's severe pain and suffering were of such great magnitude that his autonomous capacity was limited. Proponents of respect for autonomy would not be able to morally justify the preceding decision; they would argue that both Mr and Mrs J were rational and overturning their mutually agreed upon decision showed lack of respect for them as persons.

REFLECTION ON DECISION AND COURSE OF ACTION

V. Reflection on Decision and Course of Action
  A. Reflection on Decision
     1. Was the decision that was made the one that was actually acted upon? If not, why not?
     2. Did the decision that was made accomplish its intended purpose? If not, why not?
     3. In retrospect, do you believe the decision that was made was morally good or right? Why? Why not?
  B. Reflection on Course of Action
     1. Was the selected course of action carried out in the manner intended? If not, why not?
     2. Did the selected course of action accomplish its intended purpose? If not, why not?
     3. In retrospect, do you believe the course of action taken was morally good or right? Why? Why not?

The decision made by the patient and the consequent suicide did accomplish Mr J's intended purpose of death. Mr J's decision, however, was overridden by the agency lawyer who advised the Assistant Director that an unnatural death (suicide) should be prevented. It appears in this case, then, that legal considerations ultimately overrode all other considerations. One must note that this is not a desirable way to resolve *ethical* issues. That is, while the legal decision protected the hospital and its staff from possible liability, it also clearly violated the wishes of the patient and his wife. A final decision based on ethical considerations (e.g., duty of paternalism) would have provided a moral basis for overriding the patient's and his wife's wishes, if indeed the Assistant Director and her staff felt that the patient's request for autonomous suicide could not be honored.

The course of action selected by the lawyer and Assistant Director was carried out (i.e., an ambulance was called and the patient was taken to the hospital), but this action did not accomplish its intended purpose (saving of the patient's life). On the other hand Mrs J's selected course of action (cancel the ambulance and let her husband die in peace) was overridden, but, nonetheless, the outcome she desired partly occurred (her husband died, but how peacefully is unknown). The course of action taken may have been legally correct; however, one must ask whether it was morally correct as the expressed wishes of Mr and Mrs J were overridden for legal reasons. One must also ask whether a lawyer who serves as a patient advocate would have made the same legal decision as the lawyer in this case who served as the agency advocate.

CASE COMMENTARY[3]

In reviewing the analysis of this case, I find I still have a gut reaction to someone who has such intractable pain that suicide was considered an alternative. Yet given the lack of independence combined with constant pain, his choice could be intellectually understood. Even in the face of a terminal illness, suicide is unacceptable to me. I also realize I have not experienced a similar situation; therefore, I cannot positively state my reaction if such should occur to me. My thoughts are very much colored by my religious convictions

---

[3]**Case Commentary by: Ruby Van Croft, RN, MS,** Director for Special Programs, Visiting Nurse Association, Washington, D.C.

and my upbringing by my grandparents. I was taught that there is no situation that warrants suicide.

As one grows in experience and matures, it becomes evident that you are not at liberty to judge or impose your will upon another person. Even with an inner conflict, you must respond with a sense of love to support and comfort the terminally ill and their families.

The overall analysis was helpful to me. It succinctly stated the problems and situations. Seeing problems outlined by one not involved in them helps me to detach personally for short intervals. This in turn allows a less subjective examination of the problem. It also reminds me that solutions can be sought from many sources to help relieve the heavy burden of some decisions.

The outcome of the case was the death of this patient but not in the dignified manner in which the patient, family, or the agency had wished. The patient was taken to the hospital by ambulance and died there rather than at home. I am sure this was traumatic to his wife as well as our staff. On my part there was a sense of frustration and sadness because the policy could not support the family's and patient's wishes.

From the experience of this case, our agency has included sessions on suicide within the Advanced Illness Program. Staff are given the opportunity of expressing their thoughts on suicide and are also given ways of dealing with this crisis and their reactions to it. We have developed an agency policy regarding suicide and, although it can never cover all situations, it is frequently reviewed by staff, management, and legal counsel.

Summary. Three ethical principles dominate this case: the principle of autonomy (reflected in Mr J's autonomous suicide), the principle of respect for autonomy (reflected in Mrs J's support of her husband's suicide), and that part of the principle of beneficence that focuses on noninfliction of harm and prevention of harm. The case and its analysis raise questions about when and under what circumstances suicide is ever morally justified. The case also highlights a conflict between the ethical principle of respect for autonomy and the ethical principle of beneficence, as well as a conflict between law and ethics. These conflicts are analyzed using a systematic ethics decision making framework. Finally, the case analysis is reflected upon by the nurse administrator who wrote it.

We now turn our attention to a second case focusing on a conflict between the ethical principle of autonomy versus the ethical principle of beneficence. This case focuses on whether, and under what conditions, health personnel may interfere with a patient's decision to refuse medication.

CASE STUDY 2

The Psychiatric Patient Who Refused Medication[4]

During 1985, Mr R, a 45-year-old black male diagnosed as a paranoid schizophrenic, was an outpatient on convalescent leave at a major division of a large, psychiatric state hospital. Mr R was employed and functioning fairly independently in the community. He was obliged to return to the outpatient clinic approximately once monthly for medication and periodic supervision. He was not considered discharged. Mr R went to the division's Chief Nurse and stated that his treating psychiatrist prescribed prolixin I.M. for him and he'd had "all kinds of problems with it." Specifically, according to Mr R, the drug kept him from sustaining an erection, slowed his thinking, and prevented him from functioning normally around the community and at work.

Mr R continued by saying that he explained his concerns to the doctor, but the doctor insisted on Mr R taking the medication or the doctor would contact his employer. Mr R stated that the previous month when he didn't return to the outpatient clinic as scheduled for his prolixin injection, his employer told him that he couldn't work without taking his medication. Mr R then discovered that his psychiatrist had contacted his employer and told him of his refusing medication.

Since Mr R felt that he was being denied his right to refuse medication and felt pressured into complying with treatment by threats made by his doctor, he contacted the patient advocate after seeing the Chief Nurse. Mr R reminded the advocate of hospital policy concerning his right to refuse medication. It was explained to Mr R that he did have a right to refuse medication; however, it was not absolute and could be overridden by the Medical Director in an emergency situation or if considered in the patient's best interest. If he were to be involuntarily medicated, this situation would be evaluated every 60 days. Mr R stated he understood the policy; however, he insisted that he was not a danger to himself or others and that his relationships with his lady friends were just as important to

---

[4]**Case Submitted by: Ruby E. Elmore, RN, MSN,** retired; former Division Chief Nurse, Richardson Division, St. Elizabeth's Hospital, Washington, D.C., at the time this case occurred.

him as the effects of the medication and, furthermore, since he had to live in the community, what his friends thought of him was important too.

The psychiatrist was aware of the non-compliance policy as well as the policy of the hospital governing disclosure of information. The policy allows disclosure of patient information (e.g., mental stability or medication status) when a patient is on convalescent leave. A close relationship and agreement usually exists between the treatment team and the employer about procedures to be followed when intervention by health professionals or others may be necessary. There are occasions when, if the patient requests the employer *not* be advised of the patient's psychiatric status, the treatment team may honor the patient's request.

A day after Mr R's visit to the Chief Nurse, the patient advocate and patient visited the psychiatrist. In a private interview, the advocate stated Mr R's concerns to the psychiatrist along with Mr R's allegation that the psychiatrist had threatened to contact his supervisor if he refused medication. The psychiatrist responded affirmatively to Mr R's statement with the following clarifications:

1. Mr R's past history indicates that he deteriorates when not on medication.
2. Mr R's supervisor asked to be contacted when Mr R refused medication because, without medication, Mr R becomes assaultive and a potential danger to himself and others.
3. When on convalescent leave, legal measures can be used to ensure compliance to medication regimens.

At the termination of the interview, the psychiatrist refused to change or discontinue the patient's medication. The decision was based on the psychiatrist's professional judgment that the risk of Mr R's deterioration and assaultiveness outweighed the side effects of the medication. To gain support for his claim that the medication was unnecessary and that he would perform on his job without it, Mr R requested a conference with the treatment team. The treatment team concluded that:

1. They were knowledgeable of Mr R's right to refuse medication and certainly respected his right to the extent that they directed him to the patient advocate.
2. In the past when Mr R refused to take his medication, he lost his job and eventually his apartment.
3. Mr R assaulted his supervisor and was involved in several altercations when he stopped taking his medication.

At the termination of the conference, the treatment team concluded that it would be in the patient's best interest if he would accept the medication.

In a private conversation with the advocate, Mr R was asked to make a final decision about taking the prescribed psychotropic medication. Mr R stated that he would think it over and let the advocate know if he would accept the medication or refuse it voluntarily and then ask for an administrative review in accordance with hospital policy.

Mr R was later visited at his work site and asked about his decision. He stated that he decided to accept the medication under duress.

DATA COLLECTION AND ASSESSMENT

I. Data Collection and Assessment
  A. Situational Considerations
    1. What situational factors contribute to the ethical dilemma or issue?
    2. How do these situational factors contribute to the ethical dilemma or issue?
  B. Health Team Considerations
    1. What persons are most involved in the situation?
    2. What are the relevant backgrounds (e.g., educational level, value orientations) of the persons most involved?
    3. What persons are most affected by the outcome of the decision?
  C. Organizational Considerations
    1. What is the nature and mission of the organization?
    2. What are the organization's values, policies, and procedures relevant to the situation?

Situational Considerations

The situational factors contributing to the ethical dilemma, and their method of contribution, are as follows:

1. *Mr R, a psychiatric patient with outpatient status, refused to take his scheduled prolixin injection* because of problems with side effects. The underlying ethical issue is whether the patient has the right to refuse medication even when in the judgment of health professionals the treatment serves the best interests of the patient.
2. *The psychiatrist refused to change or discontinue the medication.* The underlying ethical issues arise: Does the physician have grounds for overriding the patient's right to self-determination? Do conditions surrounding the situation warrant that persuasive or manipulative, measures be used? Do legal considerations apply?
3. *Is there a danger to close friends, in the employment situation, or to the community at large* if the patient exercises his right to refuse treatment? The underlying ethical consideration is whether allowing the patient the right to self-determination (to be autonomous) interferes to the extent that harm might result to others. Put another way, does the threat of harm to others outweigh the benefit of allowing Mr R his right to self-determination?

Health Team Considerations

Persons most involved in the situation were Mr R, the psychiatrist, and the advocate. The treatment team, the employer, fellow employees, and the patient's friends were the other persons involved.

Relevant information for persons most involved include:

1. *Mr R*—Mr R is a 45-year-old black male with a diagnosis of schizophrenia disorder, paranoid type. He is an outpatient on convalescent leave living away from the hospital. He works outside the hospital environment and has held a job with one employer for at least two years. He is now followed by the outpatient clinic. He has friends in the community who are "important to him." In the past, because of lapses in medical treatment, he has become psychotic and assaultive, necessitating a return to inpatient status. Mr R has a clear and stated interest in his own state of affairs and is knowledgeable about his rights regarding medication administration. He is also mindful about working within the system.
2. *The psychiatrist*—The psychiatrist clearly explained to Mr R the necessity for continuing medication, reiterated hospital policy, restated potential consequences of non-compliance, and stated reasons for notification of Mr R's employer if the medication was not continued. The professional judgment of the psychia-

trist was that Mr R continue taking medication. Although there was difficulty in assessing the value orientation of the psychiatrist, it must be assumed that he treated the patient according to his best clinical professional judgment.

3. *The advocate*—The patient's advocate was mentioned as one of the first contacts for the patient's problems. The advocate listened, assessed, and acted to assist the patient with his complaint. Meetings were arranged by the advocate to facilitate Mr R's working through the problem. In this case, the advocate remained available and open to communication, advising the patient in a professionally competent manner.

The person most affected by the decision was Mr R as his refusal to take medication had ramifications for his continued employment and outpatient status. His employer and his friends were also affected since his medical treatment was deemed necessary for his continued stable state.

Organizational Considerations

The organization was a hospital with outpatient services for psychiatric patients such as Mr R. Like most hospitals, this bureaucratic organization operated within a particular structure having stated policies and procedures. One explicitly identified hospital policy concerns a patient's right to refuse medication and conditions under which the right might be overridden (e.g., an emergency situation or if considered in the patient's best interest), plus procedures to be followed if a patient were to be medicated involuntarily. Another policy affecting this case concerns situations in which certain information about a psychiatric patient may be disclosed. The organization has established patient advocacy policies and has a treatment team.

PROBLEM IDENTIFICATION

II. Problem Identification
   A. Ethical Considerations
      1. What are ethical considerations related to the case?
      2. Which of these ethical considerations take priority?

   B. Nonethical Considerations
     1. What are nonethical considerations related to the case (e.g.,
       medical, legal, or factual considerations)?
     2. How do the nonethical considerations relate to the ethical
       considerations?

Ethical Considerations

Major ethical considerations in the case are as follows:

1. *In regard to Mr R*—Does Mr R have the right to refuse medication? Does he have the right to be self-determining (autonomous) about this issue? Is Mr R's capacity to judge rationally
impaired by his illness?
2. *In regard to the psychiatrist*—Has the psychiatrist intervened appropriately? Should he override the patient's right to be self-
determining? In so doing, is the psychiatrist committing a
breach of confidentiality? Is he justified in using persuasion or
manipulation to accomplish what he understands to be "in the
best interests of the patient?"

Nonethical Considerations

The major nonethical consideration in this case was the hospital policy
governing the question of what was to be done in instances when
psychiatric patients refused treatment. If Mr R had insisted upon refusing treatment, legal measures may have been taken. Other nonethical
considerations revolve around Mr R's capacity to remain employed and
employable. If he is in a continued stable state, he is better prepared to
become a productive member of the community.

CONSIDERATION OF POSSIBLE ACTIONS: UTILITARIAN THINKING

III. Consideration of Possible Actions
   A. Utilitarian Thinking
     1. How is the principle of utility being defined in this case (e.g.,
       happiness, pleasure, health, etc)?

2. What are viable actions in this case?
3. What are the predicted consequences of the actions for persons affected by the decision?
4. From the predicted consequences, what is the intrinsic value and disvalue for each viable consequence?
5. What possible action(s) produce the best consequences overall for happiness, pleasure, health, etc and the least unhappiness, disvalue, displeasure, etc for persons affected, or most affected, by the decision?

Definition of the Principle of Utility

For the persons most involved in this case, the principle of utility is being applied differently. The psychiatrist and the advocate, as well as the treatment team, believed that the greatest good and the least harm would result if the patient adhered to hospital policy. In situations such as this one that involve insistence on medication compliance for mental patients, intervention may be consistent with utilitarianism. Consequences of the intervention must be examined and in certain situations, when probable benefits may result for all persons concerned, the principle would be upheld. The "most total good," however, is a moot question open to debate (Barry, 1982, pp. 339–340). For Mr R utility is being able to make his own decisions about whether or not to take his medications and to be free of the problems caused by side effects. In addition, utility for Mr R should take into consideration not harming others through assaultive behavior.

Viable Actions

Viable actions to consider in this case include the following:

1. Patient consents to take medication and returns to stable state.
2. Patient continues to refuse medication.

Predicted Consequences

For the persons most affected by the decision, predicted consequences are as follows:

	Medication accepted	Medication refused
1. For Mr R	• continued employment • continued outpatient status	• reduction of side effects • probable psychotic or assaultive behavior

	Medication accepted	*Medication refused*
	• function normally around the community • continued side effects • maintenance of stable state • loss of relationships with female friends	• return to inpatient status • loss of job • loss of fellow employees • maintain ability to sustain an erection and, thus, maintain relationships with female friends
2. *For the psychiatrist*	• conformation to hospital policy • reinforcement that the decision was a "right" decision • reinforcement for making similar future decisions	• loss of esteem in face of possible confrontation about policy • recourse to legal means • consideration of an alternate antipsychotic drug
3. *For the advocate*	• conformation to hospital policy • cessation of advocate role for Mr. R • reinforcement that the decision was a "right" decision	• loss of esteem for failure to produce a favorable outcome • potential decrease of patient trust

Intrinsic Value/Disvalue of Consequences

The primary intrinsic value of the consequences if Mr R consented to treatment was a continued stable mental state, which would allow him employment, outpatient privileges, and increased personal freedom. For the psychiatrist and the advocate the primary value was one of fulfilling the professional role within a bureaucratic system.

Outcomes of Actions Regarding Happiness/Unhappiness

For Mr R the greatest happiness would occur if he could continue to take the medication and be free of side effects. For the psychiatrist and the advocate the greatest happiness would occur only if the patient consented to treatment. We know from the outcome that the patient agreed to accept the medication under what he perceived to be duress. If the patient had not, the system would have exerted enough pressure at some point that the patient would have been compelled. Legal sanctions exist for patients like Mr R who are on convalescent leave and refuse to take medication. Hospital policy empowers the organization to notify police to pick up the patient, who is considered on "unauthorized leave status" and return him to the hospital. The patient is then returned to inpatient status with all attendant constraints and prohibitions.

CONSIDERATION OF POSSIBLE ACTIONS: DEONTOLOGICAL THINKING

III. Consideration of Possible Actions, continued
   B. Deontological Thinking
      1. What ethical rules and principles are in conflict?[5]
      2. What duties emerge from these ethical rules and principles?
      3. Which of these duties are in conflict with equal or stronger duties?
      4. If a conflict exists, which duties derived from moral rules and principles produce the greatest balance of rightness over wrongness?

Ethical Rules and Principles in Conflict

Major ethical rules and/or principles in conflict in this case are as follows:

1. *In regard to Mr R*—The principle of autonomy (i.e., Mr R was self-determining enough to make many decisions regarding his welfare) is in conflict with that aspect of the principle of beneficence that focuses on the noninfliction of harm (i.e., Mr R may cause harm to others when he insists on being self-determining).

2. *In regard to the psychiatrist*—The principle of respect for autonomy (i.e., health professionals give due appreciation to Mr R's wishes) is in conflict with those aspects of the principle of beneficence that focus on the noninfliction of harm and the duty to

---

[5]**Note:** A rule utilitarian would also raise questions about ethical rules and principles but would assess the rules in terms of consequences instead of duties.

promote good (i.e., health professionals have moral obligations to not harm and to do good). In addition for the psychiatrist, the principle of respect for autonomy is in conflict with the rule of fidelity to uphold organizational policy and procedures, although such a rule would need some moral justification.

3. *In regard to the advocate*—The principle of respect for autonomy is in conflict with the rule of fidelity to uphold organizational policy and procedures that are morally justifiable.

Duties Emerging from Rules and Principles

In this case, prima facie duties emerging from the various principles are as follows:

1. From the principle of autonomy arises the duty to act in accord with one's autonomous choices, provided the capability to make rational decisions exists.
2. From the principle of respect for autonomy arises the duty not to interfere in the autonomous choices of others, provided that autonomous choices are made rationally.
3. From the principle of beneficence arise the duties of noninfliction of harm, prevention of harm, and promotion of good.
4. From the rule of fidelity arises the duty to honor contractual or role obligations. Adherence to the rule of fidelity is not absolute, and other moral principles and rules may limit fidelity. The upholding of policies and procedures at all times may be overridden by stronger duties and obligations.

Duties in Conflict

For this case the discussion will focus on the conflict between patient autonomy and beneficence. The health professionals needed to achieve a balance between their duty not to interfere with the autonomous choices of the patient and to act with beneficence, within the bounds of their professional role obligations and responsibilities.

One could question whether the patient in this case was autonomous or had any autonomous choices at all. Let us assume that the patient possessed the capacity to act autonomously and then indeed acted autonomously, as defined in Chapter 3. The patient rationally brought the problem to the appropriate persons in an acceptable manner. Mr R even reminded the advocate of hospital policy concerning his right to refuse medication. Mr R's autonomy was compromised when he discovered that the psychiatrist had contacted his employer and told him of Mr R's refusal to take medication. Informing the employer of patient status was the normally followed procedure; however, indications are that the patient did not know this or had been told, only to forget. The facts of the case allude to Mr R's perception of the psychiatrist's communication as threatening. Such perceptions while they may be common among psychiatric patients, are also formed among healthy, mentally stable individuals.

The psychiatrist, the advocate, and the treatment team all responded similarly to the dilemma faced by the patient:

1. The health professionals knew and reinforced the stated policy about the right to refuse medication.
2. The patient's best interest would be served if he consented to treatment.

Both statements seem to conflict. On one hand, the health professionals acknowledge the patient's right to decide, and on the other, they decide what is in the patient's best interest. Overriding patients' decisions to benefit them or to prevent harm to them is paternalism (Faden & Beauchamp, 1986, p. 13). (*See* Chapter 3 on "The Problem of Paternalism.") This shall be discussed further with specific application to this case.

According to McConnell (1982, p. 77), a case may be made for justifiable treatment, with or without consent. Justifiable treatment may be used, and the patient may be persuaded or manipulated into accepting treatment, as an appeal to the harm principle. If failure to treat causes a threat of harm to self or to others, then persuading or manipulating the patient to accept treatment may be justified. A threat of harm to self or to others existed, and the psychiatrist influenced Mr R to accept treatment.

The question of influence or control impinges upon respect for autonomy of persons because fully autonomous action occurs without the controlling influence of another. According to Faden and Beauchamp (1986, pp. 261–262), influencing may range from persuasion (which is never controlling) to manipulation (which may or may not be controlling) to coercion (which is always controlling). In this instance the psychiatrist's control fell somewhere between persuasion and manipulation. In a controlled action there is a heavy measure of control, authority, and prescription (Faden & Beauchamp, 1986, p. 258). The patient perceived being threatened, and the psychiatrist had the power to carry out the threat. In other words, the wishes of the patient to be allowed to decide about his medication were overridden for what the psychiatrist thought was beneficent action, that is, using his professional judgment to decide what was for the good of the patient.

Paternalism as it relates to this case may be justified as weak paternalism because Mr R's condition, a potentially unstable state caused by his possible refusal to accept medication, might continue to deteriorate. Furthermore, other persons are at risk of harm should the lack of medication cause Mr R to become assaultive and dangerous. His psychiatric diagnosis may be indicative of diminished capacity for decision making, therefore presenting justification for the limitation of autonomous choices and making a case for weak paternalism.

Greatest Balance of Rightness over Wrongness

Provided that Mr R's psychiatric diagnosis does not interfere with his capability to make some rational decisions for himself, his moral duty is to retain decision making in regard to taking or not taking the medication. Thus his autonomy would be preserved, producing the greatest balance of rightness over wrongness. For the psychiatrist, the advocate, and the treatment team, the duty not to interfere in the autonomous choices of others and the principle of respect for autonomy would be upheld as well. The health professionals, however, have a moral duty not to do harm, which produces more rightness than their duty to not interfere with Mr R's autonomy. The decision to act in the best interests of Mr R and the other persons involved (i.e., the employer and friends) is based on the principle of beneficence to prevent harm and to do good. The decision to allow Mr R the option of choice in the matter, once all the facts were known to him, produced the greatest balance of rightness over wrongness.

DECISION AND SELECTION OF COURSE OF ACTION

IV. Decision and Selection of Course of Action
   A. Contribution of Internal/Group Factors
      1. For whom is the decision being made?
      2. Who should decide?
      3. What biases/values of persons involved in the situation affect the decision?

  B. Contribution of External Factors
    1. What institutional factors are affecting the decision and selected course of action?
    2. What legal factors are affecting the decision and selected course of action?
    3. What social factors are affecting the decision and selected course of action?
  C. Quality of Decision and Course of Action
    1. What decision is being made?
    2. What course of action to implement the decision is being made?
    3. In light of the preceding factors, is the decision being made and the course of action to be taken ones that can still be morally justified?
    4. If not, how can the decision being made and the course of action to be taken be altered so that they are morally justified?
    5. Is the selected course of action based on the decision implementable?

Contribution of Internal/Group Factors

As discussed in Chapter 4, decision making involves human judgment and choice. These processes are affected by internal and personal factors such as values and educational level.

Mr R is the focus of the decision making in this case. Health professionals acted to guide Mr R toward a decision because of his diagnosis as a psychiatric patient and his status as an outpatient. Who should make the decision is not altogether clear. Health professionals' intervention on the patient's behalf must be morally justified and ethically motivated. Simply adhering to organizational policy and procedures may not be in the patient's best interest.

Veatch (1977, p. 255) considered the unique dilemmas facing health care professionals in psychiatry and psychotherapy. In an exploration of the status of rights of "the patient to determine his own bodily destiny," the debate about free will stemming from the libertarian tradition is set forth. At the root of the problem lie two questions to be answered: (1) Are reasons present to exert influence to override the patient's right to autonomous action; and (2) are the patient's rational capabilities impaired to the point at which the decision must be made by another party? (Veatch, 1977, p. 256) The psychiatrist, the advocate, and the treatment team probably would answer the first question affirmatively. The second question needs additional data to be evaluated further.

Other values include those biases and prejudices held by the health professionals, their struggle between allegiance to the patient and to the organization, and the degree to which their jobs would be affected if a "wrong" decision was made. The treatment team conference allowed exploration of the issue. Although it is not known whether or not the problem was decided through ethical exploration of the patient's problem, the group was clear on projections of possible future events. Their experiences with similar past problems would have influenced the decision made.

Contribution of External Factors

In this case the dominant external factors were hospital policies concerning the patient's right to refuse medication, procedures set up for administrative review, and sanctions available for infractions committed by patients in convalescent leave status. Explicit guidelines were in place.. Patient status was such that policies were applicable and enforced. Legal implications were high that if any potential danger caused by the patient posed a threat, the hospital may have been placed in a position of liability.

Recent events and court decisions in New York state (Yen, 1988, p. A14) regarding homeless persons highlight problems involved in implementing policy decisions in cases of the homeless and/or mentally ill persons. Homeless person Joyce Brown was detained against her will by the City of New York and committed to Bellevue Hospital in October 1987. In November 1987 a state judge ruled that she posed no danger. She requested her own release, but the state prevailed and she remained confined. Ms Brown was released after a total of 12 weeks, in January 1988, when a state judge ruled that she could not be given medication against her will and that no cause existed for her to be detained. The New York Civil Liberties Union helped her to obtain her freedom. The test case for New York state points up problems in applying general policy and procedures to solve complex problems that have ethical and moral overtones.

Quality of Decision and Course of Action

The decision was made by the health professionals to enforce policies in effect. Justified weak paternalism with persuasion and manipulation appear to have been used to gain patient compliance. Mr R decided to accept the medication, and the problem seemed to resolve itself. What if the patient, however, had continued to refuse treatment (for whatever reason)? Would the health professionals have resorted to legal means to obtain consent to treat? How far would the persons most involved had pursued the question? Justified weak paternalism is supported in the literature (Barry, 1982; Beauchamp & Childress, 1983), but how far should it extend? When does it become unjustifiable restraint of personal autonomy?

REFLECTION ON DECISION AND COURSE OF ACTION

V. Reflection on Decision and Course of Action
   A. Reflection on Decision
      1. Was the decision that was made the one that was actually acted upon? If not, why not?
      2. Did the decision that was made accomplish its intended purpose? If not, why not?
      3. In retrospect, do you believe the decision that was made was morally good or right? Why? Why not?
   B. Reflection on Course of Action
      1. Was the selected course of action carried out in the manner intended? If not, why not?
      2. Did the selected course of action accomplish its intended purpose? If not, why not?
      3. In retrospect, do you believe the course of action taken was morally good or right? Why? Why not?

The decision to have the patient accept treatment was made and carried out by health professionals based on those aspects of the principle of beneficence to not inflict harm (or allow harm to be inflicted) and to do good in the best interest of the patient. The decision accomplished the purpose of having the patient accept treatment and seemed to have been guided by the prevailing policies. Autonomous acts by the patient were limited to the appeal process and it was clear that Mr R knew of his rights and responsibilities.

The decision was a morally right decision reflective of beneficent principles; however, the patient's perception of threat to his employment and patient status was an important factor to consider. Health professionals in this case seemed to have acted paternalistically.

In reviewing the case, it was felt that the initial question addressed by the persons involved, including Mr R, was in error. The problem here was what to do about the medication side effects. This clinical treatment problem could be solved quite easily. The moral issues explored about consent to or refusal of treatment, autonomy versus beneficence, and paternalism and control, illustrate the complexity encountered in real world situations.

CASE COMMENTARY[6]

When the patient informally discussed his case with me, he made a good presentation of his situation. He was adamant, yet rational, in his thinking about and discussion of his medication and its side effects. My first reaction was to contact the treatment team and to ask if they could give the patient a medication holiday. It was the patient's idea to go to the patient advocate to have his problem formally addressed. Consequently, I took no personal action on his part.

The case analysis highlights several ethical principles, especially the ethical principles of autonomy and respect for autonomy. Regarding the latter, psychiatric patients are no exceptions. They should be free to choose and to act without having controlling restraints placed on them by others except when they may do harm to self or others. This ethical principle is also a legal ruling applied in psychiatric settings. Inherent in the legal principle is the duty of disclosure, which the treatment team has in this case. Since failure to take medication may result in psychotic assaultive behavior, there is a duty to notify the patient's work supervisor if the patient fails to take medication.

To whom is the principle of beneficence owed—the patient, the patient's supervisor, the institution, or the community at large? If the psychotic assaultive behavior is controlled, the treatment team has provided a benefit to the patient, his supervisor, the institution, and the community by preventing harm. Insisting that the patient take medication, however, does not satisfy the principle of nonmaleficence from the patient's viewpoint because he viewed the side effects as personal harm.

---

[6]**Case Commentary by: Ruby E. Elmore, RN, MSN,** retired; Former Division Chief Nurse, Richardson Division, Saint Elizabeth's Hospital, Washington, D.C., at the time this case occurred.

This case brings to light the importance of autonomy in treatment choices. It validates the importance of being "normal." It gives emphasis to the importance of sexual virility, especially in males. It makes us more cognizant of the effects of psychotropic medications that affect the mind and physiological body functions. It is a significant psychiatric treatment issue that cannot be ignored in today's practice.

I advocate more cases of this nature for analysis and study. In-depth analysis will give treatment teams guidelines that will allow them to go beyond agonizing conflicts of wondering what to do and hoping that particular events will not happen. Yes or no answers are not readily applicable in ethical issues in psychiatric treatment.

Summary. Three ethical principles and one rule are highlighted in this case: the principle of autonomy (for the patient), the principle of respect for autonomy (for the health professionals), those aspects of the principle of beneficence that focus on noninfliction of harm and the duty to promote good, and the rule of fidelity to uphold organizational policy (explored with regard to the health professionals). The case and its analysis raise questions about when and under what circumstances health care professionals are justified in overriding patient autonomy to make decisions in the patient's best interest. Questions about paternalism and what constitutes control add substance to the analysis. Major ethical principles and rules in conflict are explicated and analyzed using a systematic ethics decision making framework. Finally, the case analysis is reflected upon by the nurse administrator who wrote it.

REFERENCES

Barry, V. (1982). *Moral aspects of health care.* Belmont, CA: Wadsworth.

Beauchamp, T. L. (1982). *Philosophical ethics: An introduction to moral philosophy.* New York: McGraw–Hill.

Beauchamp, T. L., & Childress, J. F. (1983). *Principles of biomedical ethics* (2nd ed.). New York: Oxford University Press.

Brandt, R. B. (1986). The morality and rationality of suicide. In T. A. Mappes & J. S. Zembaty (Eds.), *Biomedical ethics* (2nd ed., pp. 337–343). New York: McGraw–Hill.

Faden, R. R., & Beauchamp, T. L. (1986). *A history and theory of informed consent.* New York: Oxford University Press.

McConnell, T. C. (1982). *Moral issues in health care: An introduction to medical ethics.* Monterey, CA: Wadsworth.

Mill, J. S. (1979). *Utilitarianism* (G. Sher, Ed.). Indianapolis: Hackett. (Original work published 1861)

Veatch, R. M. (1977). *Case studies in medical ethics.* Cambridge, MA: Harvard University Press.

Veatch, R. M., & Fry, S. T. (1987). *Case studies in nursing ethics.* Philadelphia: Lippincott.

Yen, M. (1988, January 20). Homeless N.Y. woman wins release from hospital. *The Washington Post,* p. A14.

Principle of Beneficence Versus Principle of Nonmaleficence: Case Analyses

Mary Graney Trainor

All that lives must die
Passing through nature to eternity
  Shakespeare (Act I, scene ii)

In this chapter case situations faced by the Director of Nursing of a nursing center and an Assistant Vice President for Nursing at a children's hospital will be discussed. Theoretical content related to ethics, ethical theories, principles, and problem solving will be applied. Primary emphasis in these cases is a conflict between beneficence and nonmaleficence. Although in Chapter 3 the principle of beneficence incorporated the concept of nonmaleficence, in this discussion these principles will be treated separately. Beneficence is defined as the prevention of harm, the removal of harm, and the promotion of good, and nonmaleficence as the noninfliction of harm. Analysis of the cases is done by using the ethics decision framework discussed in Chapter 5. The framework is summarized as follows:

Ethics Decision Framework

I. Data Collection and Assessment
   A. Situational Considerations
   B. Health Team Considerations
   C. Organizational Considerations
II. Problem Identification
   A. Ethical Considerations
   B. Nonethical Considerations

III. Consideration of Possible Actions
  A. Utilitarian Thinking
  B. Deontological Thinking
IV. Decision and Selection of Course of Action
  A. Contribution of Internal/Group Factors
  B. Contribution of External Factors
  C. Quality of Decision and Course of Action
V. Reflection on Decision and Course of Action
  A. Reflection on Decision
  B. Reflection on Course of Action

The framework reflects categories that illustrate a useful process for decision making, but it is understood that readers may find a need for additional (or fewer) categories. Furthermore, in using the framework as a learning device, one finds that content is repeated. With practice, however, some steps may become integrated, expediting the collection of information necessary for ethical decision making.

CASE STUDY 1

Removal of Feeding Tube from a Comatose Patient[1]

Mrs W was a resident in a 200-bed nursing center from 1975 until early 1985. When admitted from a hospital to the nursing center, she was 75 years old and had a diagnosis of breast cancer with metastasis. Between June 1977 and October 1982, she was hospitalized seven times for diagnostic tests related to the cancer, a seizure disorder, urinary tract infection, and upper respiratory infection.

Mrs W, a single parent, raised three sons who expressed a great deal of loving concern for her, although none of them could provide the care she required in their homes. After she entered the nursing home, they visited her regularly and insisted she return to the hospital for treatment of each medical problem that occurred.

In October 1982 Mrs W was admitted to the hospital because of the seizure disorder. While hospitalized she experienced a cerebral vascular acci-

[1]**Case Submitted by: Beth R. Kleb, RN,** Director of Nursing, Fairfax Nursing Center, Fairfax, VA.

dent (CVA) which left her unresponsive and unable to swallow. At this time a nasogastric tube was inserted to maintain nutrition and hydration, and she returned to the nursing home with the tube in place. Her prognosis was poor, but the family refused to accept that fact.

In May 1983, seven months after her CVA, Mrs W's neurological status had not changed. She remained unresponsive but with excellent skin integrity and nutritional status. During the seven months, the sons adjusted to their mother's poor prognosis and spoke to the charge nurse about their wish for "no medical heroics" in the event of a medical emergency. A doctor's order was written to that effect.

Mrs W's condition remained stable until November 8, 1984, when she sustained a pathological fracture of the right femur while being turned in bed. She was admitted to the hospital where a cast was applied to her right leg, and she returned to the nursing home the next day.

On February 2, 1985, the sons met with their mother's physician, the Director of Nursing, and the general counsel for the nursing home to discuss the removal of the feeding tube. The sons were informed about the state's Natural Death Act and their right to withhold life-prolonging procedures due to Mrs W's irreversible condition. At that time a document was prepared reflecting the sons' decision to remove the tube, and all parties signed the document. The tube was removed later that day, and Mrs W died two days later.

Some nursing staff members expressed conflict to the Director of Nursing regarding Mrs W's right to die a natural death and the harm inflicted by removing the feeding tube. The Director of Nursing explained that staff members who disagreed with Mrs W's sons' decision could excuse themselves from Mrs W's care.

DATA COLLECTION AND ASSESSMENT

I. Data Collection and Assessment
   A. Situational Considerations
      1. What situational factors contribute to the ethical dilemma or issue?
      2. How do these situational factors contribute to the ethical dilemma or issue?
   B. Health Team Considerations
      1. What persons are most involved in the situation?
      2. What are the relevant backgrounds (e.g., educational level, value orientations) of the persons most involved?

3. What persons are most affected by the outcome of the decision?
C. Organizational Considerations
    1. What is the nature and mission of the organization?
    2. What are the organization's values, policies, and procedures relevant to the situation?

Situational Considerations

The following situational factors contribute to the ethical dilemma:

1. *Mrs W suffered a cerebral vascular accident (CVA) in October 1982.* A nasogastric tube inserted at that time maintained her nutritional status for approximately two years and four months. The underlying ethical issue is whether or not removing a feeding tube from a patient is ever morally justified and, if so, under what conditions. In particular, who can make that decision knowing that such a decision will ultimately result in the patient's death?
2. *Mrs W's three sons expressed attentive and loving concern toward their mother.* They visited her regularly and insisted on treatment for each medical problem. Seven months after Mrs W's CVA, her neurological status remained unchanged. At that time, her sons requested "no medical heroics" in the event of a medical emergency. Their subsequent request to remove the feeding tube raises several issues. Can family members request an action that will result in the patient's death? If so, under what conditions?
3. *Mrs W was receiving nursing care from the Fairfax Nursing Center.* The Director of Nursing, nursing staff, and physician were responsible for the patient's care and comfort, and to act in her best interests.

Health Team Considerations

Persons most involved in the situation were Mrs W and her sons, the physician, the Director of Nursing, legal counsel, and nursing staff who cared for the patient.

Relevant background information on the persons most involved includes:

1. *Mrs W*—Mrs W had been in the nursing center for ten years and was now 85 years old. She had been unresponsive for two years

and four months following a CVA which she experienced during hospitalization for a seizure disorder. A nasogastric tube was inserted at that time, but she remained comatose and unable to communicate. More recently, her femur fractured as she was being turned in bed. There was an increasing likelihood that other fractures would occur.

2. *Mrs W's sons*—The sons consistently gave their mother loving attention although they could not care for her in their homes. Following the CVA they had difficulty accepting her poor prognosis, but they gradually adjusted to the situation and requested "no medical heroics" in the event of a medical emergency.

3. *The physician*—Mrs W's physician was realistic about her prognosis. He saw the likelihood of additional fractures, which might cause pain and discomfort and require further hospitalizations.

4. *The Director of Nursing*—The Director had known Mrs W and the family since the time of admission. The nursing center's policy regarding the Virginia Natural Death Act guided the Director in assisting Mrs W's family with their decision to remove the feeding tube. She recognized the conflict experienced by some nursing staff members, made herself available to discuss the case, and allowed staff members who disagreed with the decision to excuse themselves from Mrs W's care.

5. *Legal counsel*—The lawyer for the nursing center was responsible to uphold Virginia's Natural Death Act. He was required to ascertain that the motives of Mrs W's sons were in the best interests of their mother.

6. *Nursing staff*—The nurses and nursing aides had cared for Mrs W over an extended period of time. They expressed their conflict regarding the harm inflicted by removing the feeding tube, thus hastening Mrs W's death.

The person most affected was Mrs W, who would die after the removal of the feeding tube. Her sons would not only experience loss but also some ambivalence about making a decision that resulted in her death. The Director of Nursing, the physician, and legal counsel were responsible to determine Mrs W's best interests and abide by state law. Some nursing staff members were troubled because of their long relationship with Mrs W. They may have felt ambivalent about caring for her, knowing that death occurred because of a decision with which they disagreed.

Organizational Considerations

The Fairfax Nursing Center had an established policy based on the Virginia Natural Death Act. This policy stipulated that residents are entitled to participate in decisions regarding the withdrawal of medical procedures that will prolong their life. In this case the organization needed to ascertain that family members made a decision that protected Mrs W's best interests.

PROBLEM IDENTIFICATION

II. Problem Identification
  A. Ethical Considerations
    1. What are ethical considerations related to the case?
    2. Which of these ethical considerations take priority?
  B. Nonethical Considerations
    1. What are nonethical considerations related to the case (e.g., medical, legal, or factual considerations)?
    2. How do the nonethical considerations relate to the ethical considerations?

Ethical Considerations

Major ethical considerations in the case are as follows:

1. *In regard to Mrs W*—Since Mrs W cannot make a decision, who decides whether removing the feeding tube, which will result in death, is in the patient's best interests?
2. *In regard to Mrs W's sons*—Should Mrs W's sons make a decision that will result in her death? If so, why?
3. *In regard to the physician, the Director of Nursing, and legal counsel*—Should they concur with the sons' request to remove the feeding tube? How can they determine which actions are most beneficial to the patient?
4. *In regard to nursing staff*—Should they continue to provide care to Mrs W if they disagreed with the decision to remove the feeding tube?

Nonethical Considerations

The major nonethical consideration was a nursing center policy that upheld the Virginia Natural Death Act. The law stipulates that competent persons diagnosed as suffering from a condition considered terminal may exercise their right to have life-prolonging procedures withdrawn. In the physician's opinion there was no hope for recovery due to the patient's medical condition, that is, irreversible coma. In addition, the likelihood of additional fractures and the possibility of subsequent pain raised further concerns about the patient's comfort. Mrs W's sons, as agent for their mother, requested removal of the feeding tube because of these concerns. In similar situations a legal guardian may be appointed, who would make decisions for the patient. Such an appointment was not considered because of the staff's long-standing relationship with the family and their trust that Mrs W's sons would act in the patient's best interests.

CONSIDERATION OF POSSIBLE ACTIONS: UTILITARIAN THINKING

III. Consideration of Possible Actions
  A. Utilitarian Thinking
    1. How is the principle of utility being defined in this case (e.g., happiness, pleasure, health, etc)?
    2. What are viable actions in the case?
    3. What are predicted consequences of the actions for persons affected by the decision?
    4. From the predicted consequences, what is the intrinsic value and disvalue for each viable consequence?
    5. What possible action(s) produce the best consequences overall for happiness, pleasure, health, etc and the least unhappiness, disvalue, displeasure, etc for persons affected, or most affected, by the decision?

Definition of the Principle of Utility

In this case the principle of utility appears to be similarly defined by the patient's three sons, the physician, the Director of Nursing, and legal counsel. Their definition sees utility as that which would maximize benefits, minimize harm, and produce freedom from pain. Mrs W's feeding tube provided no benefit except to maintain her nutritional status, which in turn increased the likelihood that she would incur additional fractures and perhaps experience pain and discomfort. For some nursing staff members, the principle of utility appears to be related to the noninfliction of harm that would hasten Mrs W's death as a result of removing the feeding tube.

Viable Actions

Viable actions to take in this case include the following:

1. Remove Mrs W's feeding tube.
2. Continue tube feedings.

The principle of utility requires that one assess the consequences of possible actions to determine their impact on the welfare of those persons affected or most affected by the action. In terms of utilitarian thinking, the argument for removing a feeding tube goes as follows: If the benefit of tube feeding will not reverse the patient's health state, that is, in this case loss of consciousness, continuing such treatment may not be in the patient's best interests and removing the feeding tube is justifiable.

Predicted Consequences

For the persons most affected by the decision, predicted consequences are as follows:

	Feeding tube removed	*Tube feedings continued*
1. *For Mrs W*	• imminent death • comfortable death[2]	• maintain life • increase the possibility of additional fractures
2. *For Mrs W's sons*	• absence of mother's presence • relief that their mother will experience no further discomfort	• continued presence of mother • knowledge that although life was maintained, health state would not

---

[2]Although this outcome remains controversial, Lynn and Childress (1983, p. 19) claim that for patients in deep and irreversible coma "nutrition and hydration do not appear to be needed or helpful, . . ."

	Feeding tube removed	Tube feedings continued
	• guilt that their decision resulted in her death	improve • continued financial burden • anguish regarding the possiblity of further fractures
3. *For Director of Nurs-ing, legal counsel, physician*	• comfort in knowing that they were meet-ing the family's request • assurance that no ad-ditional fractures and/or other medi-cal complications would occur • ambivalence about Mrs W's death	• comfort with not feeling responsible for her death • less possibility of being challenged by others (i.e., nursing staff, oth-er families, physicians, etc)
4. *For nursing staff*	• knowledge that Mrs W will die • loss of a patient they have known for a long time • possibility Mrs W may die while in their care	• maintain Mrs W's life • continue caring for her • Mrs W may incur addi-tional fractures

Intrinsic Value/Disvalue of Consequences

The primary intrinsic value for Mrs W and her sons is the assurance that there will be no further discomfort from medical complications. For the Director of Nursing, the physician, and legal counsel, the primary intrin-sic value is respect for the wishes of Mrs W's sons, who made a decision that appeared to be in their mother's best interests. For some nursing staff members the primary intrinsic value is maintenance of life.

Outcomes of Actions Regarding Happiness/Unhappiness

For Mrs W and her sons the greatest happiness would occur if she was free of further pain and discomfort. For the Director of Nursing, the physician, and legal counsel, the greatest happiness would be as-surance that Mrs W's rights were protected by the decision to remove her feeding tube. For some nursing staff members the greatest happiness would occur if tube feedings continued and Mrs W's death was not hastened.

CONSIDERATION OF POSSIBLE ACTIONS: DEONTOLOGICAL THINKING

III. Consideration of Possible Actions, continued
   B. Deontological Thinking
      1. What ethical rules and principles are in conflict?[3]
      2. What duties emerge from these ethical rules and principles?
      3. Which of these duties are in conflict with equal or stronger duties?
      4. If a conflict exists, which duties derived from moral rules and principles produce the greatest balance of rightness over wrongness?

Ethical Rules and Principles in Conflict

Major ethical rules and principles in conflict are as follows:

1. *In regard to Mrs W*—The principles of nonmaleficence, noninfliction of harm (i.e., refrain from removing the feeding tube because such action would hasten Mrs W's death), and respect for the sanctity of human life (i.e., maintain Mrs W's life by continuing the tube feeding) are in conflict with the principle of beneficence that focuses on the prevention of harm (i.e., lessen the likelihood of additional fractures and the possibility of subsequent pain by removing the feeding tube).

2. *In regard to Mrs W's sons*—The principle of beneficence that focuses on the prevention of harm (i.e., lessen the likelihood of additional fractures and subsequent pain by removing the feeding tube), is in conflict with nonmaleficence, the noninfliction of harm (i.e., refrain from removing the feeding tube because such action would hasten Mrs W's death).

---

[3]**Note:** A role utilitarian would also raise questions about ethical rules and principles but would assess the rules in terms of consequences instead of duties.

In addition, the principles of autonomy, (i.e., acting as agent for their mother) and fidelity (i.e., the implicit promise to act in their mother's best interests) are in conflict with the principle of nonmaleficence, the noninfliction of harm (i.e., refrain from removing Mrs W's feeding tube because such action would hasten her death).

3. *In regard to the Director of Nursing, the physician, and legal counsel*—The principle of beneficence that focuses on the prevention of harm (i.e., lessen the likelihood of additional fractures and the possibility of subsequent pain by removing the feeding tube) is in conflict with nonmaleficence, the noninfliction of harm (i.e., refrain from removing the feeding tube because such action would hasten Mrs W's death).

4. *In regard to nursing staff*—The principle of respect for the sanctity of life (i.e., maintain Mrs W's life by continuing the tube feeding) is in conflict with the principle of beneficence that focuses on the prevention of harm (i.e., lessen the likelihood of additional fractures and the possibility of subsequent pain by removing the feeding tube) and respect for autonomy (i.e., not to interfere with Mrs W's sons' decision).

Duties Emerging from Rules and Principles

In this case prima facie duties emerging from the various principles are as follows:

1. From the principle of nonmaleficence comes the duty not to inflict harm.
2. From the principle of beneficence arises the duty to act in a manner that prevents harm.
3. From the principle of respect for the sanctity of life arises the duty to value and preserve human life.
4. From the principle of autonomy arises the duty to act in accord with one's autonomous choices.
5. From the principle of respect for autonomy arises the duty not to interfere in the autonomous choices of others.
6. From the principle of fidelity comes the duty to keep implicit promises.

Duties in Conflict

In this case, Mrs W's sons, the physician, the Director of Nursing, and legal counsel worked through any conflicts of duty. All parties appeared motivated to protect Mrs W's best interests and conform to the legal requirement stipulated by the state's Natural Death Act.

For some nursing staff members, the conflict arose out of the duty to preserve the sanctity of life by continuing to feed Mrs W and to prevent the harm of additional fractures and the possibility of subsequent pain by removing the feeding tube. Other staff members experienced conflict with the duty to respect Mrs W's sons' autonomy to act as agent for their mother and make decisions deemed in her best interests, and the value to respect the sanctity of human life by continuing tube feedings.

Since nursing staff members were not involved in the decision and could remove themselves from the situation if they so desired, the burden of a morally justifiable decision rested with the sons, the physician, the Director of Nursing, and legal counsel.

Greatest Balance of Rightness Over Wrongness

For Mrs W's sons, the moral duty to act as autonomous agents in their mother's best interests (i.e., remove the feeding tube) and fulfill an implied promise of fidelity produced more rightness than prolonging her life by continuing the tube feedings and increasing the likelihood of additional fractures and the possibility of subsequent pain. For the Director of Nursing, the physician, and legal counsel, the moral duty to prevent further harm (i.e., lessen the likelihood of additional fractures and the possibility of subsequent pain) produced more rightness than prolonging Mrs W's life by continuing the tube feeding when there was no likelihood of improvement in her condition. For some nursing staff members the duty to preserve human life took precedence over the harm incurred by hastening her death despite the likelihood of additional fractures and subsequent pain.

DECISION AND SELECTION
OF COURSE OF ACTION

IV. Decision and Selection of Course of Action
    A. Contribution of Internal/Group Factors
        1. For whom is the decision being made?
        2. Who should decide?
        3. What biases/values of persons involved in the situation affect the decision?

B. Contribution of External Factors
   1. What institutional factors are affecting the decision and selected course of action?
   2. What legal factors are affecting the decision and selected course of action?
   3. What social factors are affecting the decision and selected course of action?
C. Quality of Decision and Course of Action
   1. What decision is being made?
   2. What course of action to implement the decision is being made?
   3. In light of the preceding factors, is the decision being made and the course of action to be taken ones that can still be morally justified?
   4. If not, how can the decision being made and the course of action to be taken be altered so that they are morally justified?
   5. Is the selected course of action based on the decision implementable?

Contribution of Internal/Group Factors

Chapter 4 states that decision making involves human judgment and choice, processes affected by internal and personal factors such as values and educational level. Mrs W is the focus of the decision making process in this case, but because she is incompetent her sons serve as proxy decision makers. Assisting them are the physician, the Director of Nursing, and legal counsel, who are responsible for determining that Mrs W's best interests are served and that the legal requirements of the state's Natural Death Act are met.

In this case who should decide seems clear. Beauchamp and Childress (1983) state that whenever possible family members should act as proxy decision makers if it can be determined that they serve the best interest of the patient. Family members established and maintained ongoing contact with the staff and insisted that Mrs W receive hospital treatment whenever necessary. The physician, however, complied with their request for "no heroics" in the event of a medical emergency. The pathological fracture incurred by simply turning her in bed and the possibility of additional fractures raised serious questions whether continued tube feedings would serve Mrs W's best interests.

Values underlying this case reflect a long standing dilemma regarding ordinary versus extraordinary or obligatory versus optional means of treatment. Some staff members saw the continued use of tube feeding as an obligatory form of treatment. Such a position is well-documented in the literature (Callahan, 1983; Derr, 1986). Proponents of this position claim that because food and fluids are universal human needs, to deny such needs is vastly different from the denial of medical or surgical therapies. To withhold or starve can never convey care. Others (Annas, 1986; Lynn & Childress, 1983; Paris, 1986) point out that intravenous or gastric feedings need to be evaluated on the basis of the proportionate benefit and burden they confer on the patient. Mrs W's condition was irreversible, and to maintain nutrition would only increase the possibility of additional fractures and subsequent pain.

Another value included the need to remain within the law as stipulated by the state's Natural Death Act. In addition, the Director of Nursing showed respect for staff members by allowing them not to care for Mrs W if they experienced conflict with the decision to remove the feeding tube.

Contribution of External Factors

In this case, legal and ethical considerations were congruent and the state's Natural Death Act gave guidelines for decision making to the principals involved. Mrs W's condition was irreversible with no hope for recovery, and a previous decision precluded any use of heroic measures. A long-standing relationship with the family allowed the physician, legal counsel, and the Director of Nursing to ascertain that the sons' motivation served Mrs W's best interests. No legal problems existed. Statutes vary, however, and in some states family members may not make decisions to discontinue nutrition and hydration. If appointing a legal guardian had been deemed necessary, Mrs W's life would have been extended for a protracted period of time while the courts debated the case. Such debate supposedly protects the patient's rights because she cannot speak for herself; however, Mrs W would have been subjected to the likelihood of additional fractures and the possibility of subsequent pain. This case did not present a conflict between ethical and moral considerations, but in many situations this conflict becomes problematic and creates great distress for those involved. In such situations one must ask if legal sanctions uphold or violate moral principles.

Quality of Decision and Course of Action

The decision was made to remove Mrs W's feeding tube. A meeting with the patient's sons, the physician, legal counsel, and the Director of

Nursing offered the principals involved an opportunity to explore their concerns. Ultimately, the sons made a decision that they believed would serve the patient's best interests, and, after signing the necessary document, the tube was removed. Nursing staff members were allowed to express their disagreement with the decision and were excused from providing care to Mrs W if they wished. Decisions to withdraw nutrition and hydration from incompetent patients remain highly controversial. In this case the decision, based on that aspect of beneficence to prevent harm, was morally justified because of the patient's irreversible condition and the likelihood of additional fractures, and the possibility of subsequent pain, and discomfort.

REFLECTION ON DECISION AND COURSE OF ACTION

V. Reflection on Decision and Course of Action
   A. Reflection on Decision
      1. Was the decision that was made the one that was actually acted upon? If not, why not?
      2. Did the decision that was made accomplish its intended purpose? If not, why not?
      3. In retrospect, do you believe the decision that was made was morally good or right? Why? Why not?
   B. Reflection on Course of Action
      1. Was the selected course of action carried out in the manner intended? If not, why not?
      2. Did the selected course of action accomplish its intended purpose? If not, why not?
      3. In retrospect, do you believe the course of action taken was morally good or right? Why? Why not?

The patient's feeding tube was removed. With no hope for recovery and the likelihood of additional fractures and the possibility of subsequent pain, Mrs W's sons, the Director of Nursing, legal counsel, and the physician acted in the patient's best interest. The decision was morally good, although Mrs W's death was hastened. Any decision to withhold nutrition and hydration from incompetent patients is disturbing, and this case reflected the current concern that such decisions must be made cautiously.

The selected course of action was carried out, and Mrs W died two days after her feeding tube was removed. The action was morally correct because the relevant consideration, based on that aspect of beneficence to prevent harm, guided a careful and deliberative decision making process directed toward the patient's benefit. In addition, staff members who disagreed with the decision were given the option to be excused from caring for the patient, thus preventing any compromise of their beliefs regarding the sanctity of life.

CASE COMMENTARY[4]

Struggles about this case had been occurring for a long time. I had known Mrs W since she entered the nursing center and was involved with the family throughout all stages of her illness. Each time that she went to a hospital for treatment, I felt badly. After the stroke, I sometimes thought that she was being "overtreated," particularly when aggressive treatment was used. Although the family requested hospitalization for each medical problem, I believed the patient would have felt better if she remained in the nursing center. Yet, Mrs W's sons needed the freedom to make decisions about their mother's care. When the family finally decided to remove Mrs W's feeding tube, I felt comfortable with their choice. The preceding analysis highlights the conflict involved and clearly reflects the difficulty of the decision.

Mrs W died peacefully within 48 hours after the tube was removed. All staff members cared for her. An important outcome was that Mrs W died within a relatively short period of time. Had she lingered, staff members would have needed more support and perhaps some staff would have taken the option not to care for her. Another critical part of the case was the Virginia Natural Death Act, which we followed to the letter of the law.

The final outcome was positive for everyone involved. Nursing staff, who initially felt badly about the decision, were actively involved in Mrs W's care until she died. With future cases of this kind the starting point is the same. Shortly after admission to the nursing center, the resident and/or family members are informed about their rights to decision making regarding treatment. We provide information about the Virginia Natural Death Act, living wills, whether cardiopulmonary resuscitation will be instituted, and the circum-

---

[4]Case Commentary by: Beth R. Kleb, RN, Director of Nursing, Fairfax Nursing Center, Fairfax, VA.

stances for discontinuing certain forms of treatment. As a result, making decisions in crisis situations is avoided. In addition, we allow staff members to make choices about whether they will care for patients when decisions about such care conflict with their ethical standards.

Summary. This case discusses the conflict between nonmaleficence, the noninfliction of harm (i.e., refrain from removing Mrs W's feeding tube because such action would hasten her death) and that aspect of beneficence to prevent harm (i.e., lessen the likelihood of additional fractures and the possibility of subsequent pain by removing the feeding tube). Another conflict exists between the principle of respect for autonomy (i.e., support the decision of Mrs. W's sons) and respect for the sanctity of life (i.e., maintain Mrs W's life by continuing the tube feeding). The case and its analysis raise questions about when and under what circumstances the withholding of nutrition and fluids is morally justifiable. An ethics decision making framework is used to guide an analysis of the conflicts, and the nurse administrator involved in the case reflects upon its resolution.

CASE STUDY 2

The Terminally Ill Dying Child[5]

Mrs M was the Director of Nursing in a 250-bed children's hospital. Ms B stopped at her office door saying, "I have to talk with you. I can't sleep at night thinking about what might happen to Jane." Ms B was a knowledgeable, experienced Unit Leader, respected by peers, staff, physicians, and administrators. She began to talk about Jane who was well known to the staff on Ms B's unit. Together they had waged a five year battle with cancer that was originally found on Jane's vocal cords and had spread throughout her body. Numerous hospitalizations involving surgery, chemotherapy and/or radiation induced remissions, and relief from pain had led to discharge. Now at age 12,

---

[5]**Case Submitted by: Jacqueline Muir, RN, MSN,** Assistant Vice President for Nursing and Operations (formerly Director of Nursing, inpatient services) Children's Hospital National Medical Center, Washington, D.C.

Jane was admitted for the last time. No medical therapies were planned, only intermittent relief from pain was possible, and there was no hope for discharge.

Ms B explained the difficulty of this last admission on the patient, family, doctors, and nurses, who knew the end was near. She described a widespread sense of failure and helplessness among those involved. They had mixed feelings of wanting Jane's life prolonged, a desire for the suffering to end, and concerns about how they might react to pleas from the patient and family. Ms B said, "I'm afraid someone will take this matter into their own hands." The child was receiving a continuous high dosage morphine drip and had been drifting in and out of consciousness for five days. The least movement of her body caused additional pain, and she was pleading with staff to "don't touch me, do something for the pain, let me die. . ."

Ms B described the moral conflict she perceived. How can we care for Jane when every movement inflicts additional pain? She no longer will eat, and tube feedings have provoked vomiting and additional pain. She is currently receiving hyperalimentation because not feeding her is also harmful. The medication is solely for pain relief, but her tolerance has escalated to the point that usually lethal doses are ineffective. Nurses are fearful that the next administered dose will cause her death. How can we justify and still control the medication administration? Where is the line between "too much is kind but harmful" and "too little is cruel but safe?" Don't we owe Jane a peaceful death? Doesn't she have the right to decide?

Mrs M discussed the issues with other unit staff members to confirm Ms B's perceptions of the dilemma. She recounted their concerns with the Medical Director. Mrs M called a patient care conference for the nurses and physicians involved and invited consultants with expertise in ethics. Participants described their worst fears, and ethical rights and duties were addressed. As a result, staff members began operating with the same knowledge regarding the patient's past medical treatments and results, current condition, and future outcomes. Algorithms were developed to address expected and unexpected events. For example, if Jane lives another five days, what medication will she be receiving? As a result, staff and family provided supportive care to one another as well as to the patient when she died 48 hours later.

DATA COLLECTION AND ASSESSMENT

I. Data Collection and Assessment
  A. Situational Considerations
    1. What situational factors contribute to the ethical dilemma or issue?

2. How do these situational factors contribute to the ethical dilemma or issue?
B. Health Team Considerations
   1. What persons are most involved in the situation?
   2. What are the relevant backgrounds (e.g., educational level, value orientations) of the persons most involved?
   3. What persons are most affected by the outcome of the decision?
C. Organizational Considerations
   1. What is the nature and mission of the organization?
   2. What are the organization's values, policies, and procedures relevant to the situation?

Situational Considerations

The following situational factors contribute to the ethical dilemma:

1. *Jane*—Jane is in the final stage of a terminal illness and experiencing excruciating pain. The underlying ethical issue is whether to comply with a 12-year-old patient's plea to be left alone and allowed to die. Under what conditions can administering potentially lethal doses of pain-relieving medication be considered as beneficial?
2. *Nursing and medical staff*—The underlying ethical issue for physicians and nursing staff is whether or not administering potentially lethal doses of pain-relieving medication and complying with a patient's request to be left alone can be morally justified. If so, under what conditions?
3. *Jane's parents*—The underlying issue for the parents is whether to comply with their daughter's wish to die and as her legal guardian request the administration of doses of medication that will relieve her pain but may also cause her death. In addition, can they support Jane's plea to be left alone and request the withholding of routine care, hydration, and nourishment?

Health Team Considerations

Persons most involved in the situation were Jane, her parents, nurses, physicians, and the Director of Nursing.

Relevant background on the persons most involved includes:

1. *Jane*—For five years Jane fought a battle with cancer that subsequently spread throughout her body. Numerous hospitaliza-

tions involving surgery, chemotherapy and/or radiation resulted in remissions, relief from pain, and ultimately discharge.
Now, at age 12, Jane was admitted to the hospital for the last
time without hope of returning home. No medical therapies
were planned, and only intermittent pain relief seemed possible. She would no longer eat, and tube feedings provoked
vomiting and caused additional pain. She was receiving hyperalimentation. Although a continuous high dosage morphine
drip was administered and she had been drifting in and out of
consciousness for five days, her tolerance had escalated to the
point that usually lethal doses were ineffective. Jane pleaded
with the staff not to touch her, to alleviate her pain, and to allow
her to die.

2. *Jane's parents*—Jane's parents knew that their daughter was
going to die, although they wanted to take her home. They had
enormous trust in the staff and relied on them to make decisions in their daughter's best interest.

3. *Nursing and medical staff*—Over the past five years, Jane had
greatly endeared herself to the staff, who described her as a
mature 12-year-old and knowledgeable about her condition.
Staff members were ambivalent about Jane's impending death
and wavered between wanting to prolong her life and a desire
for the suffering to end. They believed that not feeding her was
harmful, and they were also fearful that the next dose of medication would cause her death. Nurses wanted Jane to die peacefully and questioned whether she had a right to decide what
happened to her. Nurses and physicians believed in the hospital's philosophy regarding sanctity of life and the need to preserve life, which meant that routine care, nutrition, and hydration needed to be maintained.

4. *Mrs M*—The Director of Nursing confirmed the perceptions of
the Unit Leader and called a patient care conference. She invited the principal nursing and medical staff members involved in
Jane's care and consultants with expertise in ethics. Mrs M was
in a position of trying to assist the staff to make decisions that
would uphold the hospital's philosophy regarding sanctity of
life yet keep the patient comfortable.

The person most affected by the decision was Jane, who was entitled to a peaceful death. Her parents were troubled by the impending
loss of a child and the struggle of watching her suffer and plead to die.
Nursing and medical staff were in conflict because administering increasingly high doses of pain-relieving medication might cause her

death. They faced a dilemma: to respect the sanctity of life and also support Jane's request to die.

Organizational Considerations

The goal of Children's Hospital is to give the highest quality of medical and nursing care to patients and their families. Dying children and their families are provided with the resources necessary for a comfortable and peaceful death. The institution believes that withholding hydration, nourishment, and routine care violates respect for the sanctity of human life.

PROBLEM IDENTIFICATION

II. Problem Identification
  A. Ethical Considerations
    1. What are ethical considerations related to the case?
    2. Which of these ethical considerations take priority?
  B. Nonethical Considerations
    1. What are nonethical considerations related to the case (e.g., medical, legal, or factual considerations)?
    2. How do the nonethical considerations relate to the ethical considerations?

Ethical Considerations

Major ethical considerations in the case are as follows:

1. *In regard to Jane*—Should Jane receive increasingly high doses of pain-relieving medication that might cause her death? Should she be allowed to refuse nourishment, hydration, and routine care?
2. *In regard to Jane's parents*—Should Jane's parents, as her legal guardians, request increasingly high doses of medication that will alleviate Jane's pain but may also cause her death? In addition, should they support Jane's desire to be left alone and request the withholding of nutrition?

3. *In regard to nursing and medical staff*—Should nurses and physicians administer increasingly high doses of pain-relieving medication that may also cause her death? Should they comply with her request to be left alone and withhold routine care, nourishment, and hydration?

4. *In regard to the Director of Nursing*—How can Mrs M assist the staff to deal with administering medication that will alleviate Jane's pain but may also cause her death? Should she encourage the staff to comply with the patient's request to be left alone?

Nonethical Considerations

The major nonethical consideration was whether to comply with the patient's wishes although she was a minor. Jane's parents relinquished decision making to the staff. As a result of Jane's numerous hospitalizations, the parents trusted nurses and physicians to make decisions in their daughter's best interest. With longstanding relationships, such trust is not unusual. Staff members understood the difficulties that Jane's parents were experiencing, accepted the decision making responsibility and, in effect, became Jane's agent.

CONSIDERATION OF POSSIBLE ACTIONS: UTILITARIAN THINKING

III. Consideration of Possible Actions
   A. Utilitarian Thinking
      1. How is the principle of utility being defined in this case, (e.g., happiness, pleasure, health, etc)?
      2. What are viable actions in the case?
      3. What are predicted consequences of the actions for persons affected by the decision?
      4. From the predicted consequences, what is the intrinsic value and disvalue for each viable consequence?
      5. What possible action(s) produce the best consequences overall for happiness, pleasure, health, etc and the least unhappiness, disvalue, displeasure, etc for persons affected, or most affected, by the decision?

Definition of the Principle of Utility

In this case the principle of utility is defined slightly differently by the various persons involved. For Jane the principle of utility is defined as freedom from pain and being allowed to die peacefully. For Jane's parents the principle of utility is similarly defined, that is, alleviating the pain of seeing their daughter suffer. For nurses, physicians, and the Director of Nursing, the principle of utility is defined as being assured that their actions will contribute to the patient's welfare. In this case, welfare is defined as that which contributes to the patient's physical and psychological comfort and, insofar as possible, keeps her free of pain.

Viable Actions

In this case viable actions include the following:

1. Continue to administer nourishment, hydration, and routine care and increase the dosage of pain-relieving medication so that the patient is pain free.
2. Continue to administer nourishment, hydration, and routine care and exercise caution when administering pain-relieving medication.

In order to uphold the principle of utility, one must assess the consequences of actions to determine their impact on the welfare of those persons affected by the action. Although the administration of analgesics may hasten a person's death, the value of pain relief is greater than the harm incurred by allowing a terminally ill person to suffer excruciating pain.

Predicted Consequences

For the persons most affected by the decision, predicted consequences are as follows:

	Medication increased	*Medication cautiously administered*
1. *For Jane*	• pain relief • hasten her death • more peaceful death	• continued pain • extension of life
2. *For parents*	• relief from anguish of seeing daughter suffer • hasten loss of their daughter	• anguish in seeing their daughter suffer • additional time with their daughter

	Medication increased	Medication cautiously administered
3. For nursing and medical staff	• comfort in seeing patient experience less pain • knowledge that medication is hastening patient's death	• distress of seeing patient suffer • assurance that one's actions are not causing patient's death

Intrinsic Value/Disvalue of Consequences

The primary intrinsic value expressed by Jane is freedom from pain and a peaceful death. The primary intrinsic value for Jane's parents is love for their daughter and trusting the staff to make a decision in her best interest. For the nurses, physicians, and the Director of Nursing, the primary intrinsic value is providing care that will keep Jane pain free yet not harm her.

Outcomes of Actions Regarding Happiness/Unhappiness

For Jane and her parents, the greatest happiness would occur if she was free of pain and allowed to die a peaceful death. For the nursing and medical staff, the greatest happiness would occur if their care kept Jane free of pain and discomfort and gave her some control over her death. For the Director of Nursing, the greatest happiness would occur if she helped the staff to develop a plan of care for Jane that would keep her pain free and uphold the hospital's philosophy to value and respect human life.

CONSIDERATION OF POSSIBLE ACTIONS: DEONTOLOGICAL THINKING

III. Consideration of Possible Actions, continued
   B. Deontological Thinking
      1. What ethical rules and principles are in conflict?[6]
      2. What duties emerge from these ethical rules and principles?

[6]**Note:** A rule utilitarian would also raise questions about ethical rules and principles but would assess the rules in terms of consequences instead of duties.

3. Which of these duties are in conflict with equal or stronger duties?
4. If a conflict exists, which duties derived from moral rules and principles produce the greatest balance of rightness over wrongness?

Ethical Rules and Principles in Conflict

Major ethical rules and/or principles in conflict in this case are as follows:

1. *In regard to Jane*—The principle of respect for autonomy (i.e., respecting Jane's wishes to be left alone) is in conflict with respect for the sanctity of life (i.e., providing nutrition and hydration that will maintain her life). In addition, the principle of nonmaleficence, the noninfliction of harm (i.e., refrain from administering dosages of pain-relieving medication that might hasten her death) is in conflict with that aspect of beneficence to remove harm (i.e., alleviate pain).
2. *In regard to Jane's parents, nursing and medical staff, and the Director of Nursing*—The principle of nonmaleficence, the noninfliction of harm (i.e., refrain from administering pain-relieving medication that might hasten her death) is in conflict with that aspect of beneficence to remove harm (i.e., alleviate pain). In addition, the principle of respect for autonomy (i.e., Jane's wishes for staff to leave her alone) is in conflict with respect for the sanctity of life (i.e., maintain life by providing nutrition and hydration).

Duties Emerging from Rules and Principles

In this case, prima facie duties emerging from the various principles are as follows:

1. From the principle of respect for autonomy arises the duty not to interfere in the autonomous choices of others.
2. From the principle of beneficence arises the duty to remove harm.
3. From the principle of respect for the sanctity of life arises the duty to value and preserve human life.
4. From the principle of nonmaleficence arises the duty not to inflict harm.

Duties in Conflict

In this case the major conflict seemed to be with the nurses and the Director of Nursing who experienced the following conflict of prima facie duties:

> A conflict between the duty to respond to a terminally ill, suffering child's plea to be free of pain and be allowed to die, and the duty to preserve the sanctity of human life through the noninfliction of and removal of harm.

Since the Unit Leader turned to her administrator for help, the burden of a morally justifiable decision rested with the Director of Nursing. She was ultimately responsible for seeing that patients received the highest quality of nursing care while upholding the hospital's philosophy to respect, value, and preserve human life.

Greatest Balance of Rightness Over Wrongness

Because of her age and physical condition, Jane's autonomy was compromised, and she was forced to rely on others to carry out her wishes. For Jane's parents, the moral duty to respect their daughter's wishes was delegated to the staff. Their willingness to delegate was based on a long-standing, trusting relationship with staff members, whom the parents believed would make decisions in their daughter's best interest. For nurses, physicians, and the Director of Nursing, the moral duty to value human life produced more rightness than the duty to act according to the patient's wishes. Their belief in the sanctity of life was reflected in the continuation of nourishment, hydration, and routine care which took precedence over the patient's wishes to be left alone. The decision to keep the patient pain free was based on that aspect of beneficence to remove harm and also to respect the patient's wishes for comfort.

DECISION AND SELECTION OF COURSE OF ACTION

IV. Decision and Selection of Course of Action
    A. Contribution of Internal/Group Factors
        1. For whom is the decision being made?
        2. Who should decide?

    3. What biases/values of persons involved in the situation affect the decision?

B. Contribution of External Factors
    1. What institutional factors are affecting the decision and selected course of action?
    2. What legal factors are affecting the decision and selected course of action?
    3. What social factors are affecting the decision and selected course of action?

C. Quality of Decision and Course of Action
    1. What decision is being made?
    2. What course of action to implement the decision is being made?
    3. In light of the preceding factors, is the decision being made and the course of action to be taken ones that can still be morally justified?
    4. If not, how can the decision being made and the course of action to be taken be altered so that they are morally justified?
    5. Is the selected course of action based on the decision implementable?

Contribution of Internal/Group Factors

In this case, Jane is unable to act for herself, and her parents firmly believe that the staff will make decisions in their daughter's best interest. This trust developed during the past five years that Jane, her parents, and staff members fought a battle with cancer. Scheduling a patient care conference allowed the principals involved to express their fears and conflicts, and consultants with expertise in ethics assisted the staff to resolve these difficulties. Staff members reaffirmed their belief in the sanctity of human life and the responsibility to alleviate Jane's suffering.

Contribution of External Factors

The hospital's philosophy regarding sanctity of life stipulated that routine care, nourishment, and hydration needed to be maintained. Such a policy concurs with the position by Callahan (1983) and Derr (1986) that identifies food as a basic universal need that should not be withheld even when artificially administered. The staff strongly agreed with the hospital's position, therefore discontinuing nutrients and fluids was not a consideration. Since Jane's parents implicitly relinquished their responsibility for decision making, staff members acted as agent for the patient and focused primarily on concerns regarding the administration of pain-relieving medication.

Quality of Decision and Course of Action

The staff decided to use algorithms to guide their decisions about medication. By examining the present situation and projecting what might occur in the future, they were able to determine and anticipate the increased dosage of pain-relieving medication needed to keep Jane comfortable. As a result, nurses and physicians functioned with the same knowledge and agreed to the amount of medication that the patient might ultimately receive. This information reassured staff members and allowed them to care for Jane without compromising their values for the respect and maintenance of human life. The decision to increase the medication was morally justifiable and reflected attempts to bridge the conflict between nonmaleficence, not to inflict harm, and that aspect of beneficence to remove harm.

The possibility of withholding hydration and nutrition was not considered because of the hospital's philosophy regarding sanctity of life. Due to heightened interest in this issue, one can raise legitimate questions to determine if there are exceptions to such a position. In this case, was Jane's dying prolonged? Current debate to withhold nutrition and hydration will continue. Food and water constitute life's basic substances, and human beings are entitled to these provisions. Who should decide to withhold such substances and under what circumstances? In this situation, because of complete trust in the staff, parents of a 12-year-old child relinquished their decision making. Staff members anguished about Jane's life and death and made choices that they genuinely believed were morally correct and in her best interest. A recent series edited by Lynn (1986) provides the most comprehensive and authoritative thinking about this problem. Currently science lacks empirical data on the discomfort that results from discontinuing nutrition and hydration. Previously held beliefs asserted that hydration to maintain electrolyte balance and nutrition to prevent the effects of starvation were essential to the patient's comfort; however, hospice nurses offer information (Schmitz & O'Brien, 1986) that questions such assumptions. In some situations withholding nutrition and hydration may produce comfort and contribute to a more peaceful death. Such choices must always be made carefully and cautiously, particularly when patients cannot make their own decisions.

**REFLECTION ON DECISION
AND COURSE OF ACTION**

V. Reflection on Decision and Course of Action
   A. Reflection on Decision
     1. Was the decision that was made the one that was actually acted upon? If not, why not?
     2. Did the decision that was made accomplish its intended purpose? If not, why not?
     3. In retrospect, do you believe the decision that was made was morally good or right? Why? Why not?
   B. Reflection on Course of Action
     1. Was the selected course of action carried out in the manner intended? If not, why not?
     2. Did the selected course of action accomplish its intended purpose? If not, why not?
     3. In retrospect, do you believe the course of action taken was morally good or right? Why? Why not?

The decision to use algorithms was acted on, and Jane received the increasing doses of medication required to alleviate her pain. This decision was morally correct and congruent with the institution's beliefs regarding the sanctity of life. Acting in Jane's behalf, staff members focused on resolving the conflict between the noninfliction of harm, (i.e., refrain from administering dosages of pain-relieving medication that might cause her death) and that aspect of beneficence to remove harm (i.e., alleviation of Jane's pain). Withholding of fluids and nutrients was not considered as a possible option because of the hospital's philosophy regarding the sanctity of life. In similar cases, this issue needs further exploration to determine whether maintaining life is in the patient's best interest.

The course of action to administer medication based on algorithms was carried out. Jane received the medication required to alleviate pain and died peacefully 48 hours later. Actions focused primarily on pain relief and were morally justifiable in resolving the conflict between the noninfliction and removal of harm. One must ask, however, whether in this case withholding fluids and nutrition may have shortened the dying process and allowed Jane to be more comfortable. In future situations of this kind, one sees the need to debate the issues regarding sanctity of life, nonmaleficence, and beneficence, and consider the possibility of a cautious deliberative decision to discontinue nutrition and hydration.

CASE COMMENTARY[7]

This case points out the powerful emotional effects of caring for the dying child and demonstrates the need for caregivers to acknowledge and examine those effects. The nursing administrator can facilitate the process needed to clarify the understanding of caregivers, the patient, and family members in relation to prescribed medical therapies and pending death. The process will serve the important function of establishing a framework complete with common understanding and shared vocabulary, which will lead to elimination of miscommunication and misconceptions and promote the identification of true conflicts in values.

The preceding analysis provides many ethical principles and rules that can be applied to this case and provides a comprehensive framework that can be used by caregivers facing similar dilemmas in the future.

The caregivers involved in this case expressed their satisfaction that the issues had been addressed and misconceptions identified and clarified. Subsequent ethical dilemmas have resulted in similar meetings. In addition, the hospital's Institutional Ethics Committee has provided a forum for dilemmas that cannot be resolved at a lower level.

The philosophy of the hospital reflects the ethical traditions of the health care profession and the obligation to provide care, respect life, and "do no harm" to the patient. This philosophy is reflected in policies and procedures that provide guidelines for caregivers. Such policies and procedures are also discussed and examined freely in ethical dilemmas. The sincerely held ethical principles of caregivers and those reflected in the hospital's philosophy are usually congruent, but, when there is disagreement, a more formalized process allows thorough discussion and examination. Decisions related to continuation of hydration and nutrition are also carefully examined.

---

[7]Case Commentary by: Jacqueline Muir, RN, MSN, Assistant Vice President for Nursing and Operations (formerly Director of Nursing–Inpatient Services), Children's Hospital National Medical Center, Washington, D.C.

Summary. The major principles discussed in this case include the principle of nonmaleficence, not to inflict harm (i.e., refrain from administering dosages of pain-relieving medication that might cause Jane's death) and that aspect of beneficence to prevent harm (i.e., alleviation of pain). The case and its analysis raised questions about when administering increasingly lethal doses of medication is morally justifiable. In addition, staff's commitment to the hospital's philosophy regarding respect for the sanctity of life (i.e., maintaining life) posed a conflict with regard to respect for the patient's autonomy (i.e., respecting Jane's wishes to be left alone). In other situations, as noted in the first case analysis, staff members may face the dilemma of making decisions to discontinue or withhold nutrition and hydration. Debate about this issue continues. A decision making framework was used to analyze and resolve the conflicts and the analysis is commented on by the nurse administrator who experienced them.

REFERENCES

Annas, G. (1986). Do feeding tubes have more rights than patients? *Hastings Center Report, 16*(1), 26–28.

Beauchamp, T. L., & Childress, J. F. (1983). *Principles of biomedical ethics* (2nd ed.). New York: Oxford University Press.

Callahan, D. (1983). On feeding the dying. *Hastings Center Report, 13*(5), 22.

Derr, P. (1986). Why food and fluids can never be denied. *Hastings Center Report, 16*(1), 28–30.

Lynn, J. (Ed.). (1986). *By no extraordinary means: The choice to forgo life-sustaining food and water.* Bloomington: Indiana University Press.

Lynn, J., & Childress, J. F. (1983). Must patients always be given food and water? *Hastings Center Report, 13*(5), 17–21.

Paris, J. J. (1986). When burdens of feeding outweigh benefits. *Hastings Center Report, 16*(1), 30–32.

Schmitz, P., & O'Brien, M. (1986). Observations on nutrition and hydration in dying cancer patients. In J. Lynn (Ed.), *By no extraordinary means: The choice to forgo life-sustaining food and water* (pp. 29–38). Bloomington: Indiana University Press.

Principle of Justice Versus Principle of Beneficence: Case Analyses

Doreen Connor Harper

Justice is truth
in action.
Benjamin Disraeli

In this chapter, theoretical content related to the principle of justice is applied to actual case situations encountered by a military nurse administrator on an overseas assignment and by a nurse administrator in the Mid-Atlantic region. Both of these cases focus on the interplay between the principle of justice and the principle of beneficence to assure the "fair" distribution of resources. Although other ethical principles and issues exist, and some are touched upon, justice is emphasized as the primary ethical principle. Using the ethics decision framework discussed in Chapter 5, ethical issues in these cases will be identified and discussed in relation to ethical theories, principles, and moral values. This framework is summarized as follows:

Ethics Decision Framework

I. Data Collection and Assessment
   A. Situational Considerations
   B. Health Team Considerations
   C. Organizational Considerations
II. Problem Identification
   A. Ethical Considerations
   B. Nonethical Considerations
III. Consideration of Possible Actions
   A. Utilitarian Thinking
   B. Deontological Thinking

IV. Decision and Selection of Course of Action
   A. Contribution of Internal/Group Factors
   B. Contribution of External Factors
   C. Quality of Decision and Course of Action
V. Reflection on Decision and Course of Action
   A. Reflection on Decision
   B. Reflection on Course of Action

| CASE STUDY 1 |

Allocation of Scarce Resources in a Neonatal Intensive Care Unit[1]

As the Director of Nursing in the Army Medical Center in Frankfurt, Germany, Colonel A managed nursing operations for a 350-bed hospital. The Army Medical Center provides health care to Army personnel and their families stationed in the European command. The Center also has several intensive care units that serve all branches of the military in the European command. The most notable of these is the Neonatal Intensive Care Unit (NICU), the only neonatal center in the European command. The NICU is known for its well-qualified staff of neonatalogists and neonatal nurses. Within the military medical command, this NICU has earned its reputation based on its successful outcomes with neonates and their families.

While reviewing the incoming mail one morning, Colonel A discovered a memo from the Civilian Personnel Officer, Mr L. The memo contained a directive that all civilian personnel who had been assigned in West Germany for more than five years would be processed for return to the United States within the next 60 days. Colonel A was stunned because over one half of the professional nursing staff at the Center were civilian nurses. As she further considered the problems associated with this directive she remembered that 20 of the nurses assigned to the NICU were civilian personnel, and at least 15 of these nurses had been on the unit for five or more years.

Colonel A contacted Mr L to explain the problems that would result from implementing this policy immediately. Since the acuity level on the NICU was very high, qualified and experienced nurses were needed to provide care on the unit. By implementing this policy, virtually two-thirds of the neonatal nursing staff would be relieved of their duty on the NICU. Mr L made it clear to

---

[1]**Case Submitted by: Brigadier General Clara Adams-Ender, RN, MS, MMAS,** Chief, United States Army Nurse Corps, Washington, D.C.

Colonel A that he had no control of the situation; he perceived himself as bound by these orders. Mr L explained that the directive was due to financial cuts in the Department of Defense budget, particularly in the areas of civilian personnel and funding for overseas assignments. The civilian nurses in question had longevity and, therefore, higher salaries and benefits. Replacement of the civilian personnel with longevity by newly hired civilians could reduce the budget significantly during the next fiscal year.

Colonel A had no choice but to return civilian personnel to the United States. Colonel A made the case that the policy would essentially wipe out the nursing staff in the NICU, limiting care for the neonates and their families, but Mr L held firm to the implementation of the policy. Knowing that this policy had the potential to affect the safety of the patients on the NICU led Colonel A to consult with the Medical Center Commander, Colonel T.

Colonel A apprised Colonel T of the situation and how the directive would have a potentially life-threatening impact on the provision of nursing services in the NICU. Colonel A also pointed out that reassignment of the best NICU nurses and curtailment of services could lead to a politically sensitive situation for the Army. Colonel T agreed with Colonel A regarding the seriousness of the decision to implement this policy. Despite his concern over the effect of this policy on the safety of the neonates in the NICU, Colonel T chose to support Mr L's decision to abide by orders. He made it clear that neither did he have the power to change the policy, since it was related to budgetary constraints and clearly was a directive from a higher command, nor did he intend to risk his position by questioning these orders.

Colonel A decided to hold fast to her conviction that releasing the civilian personnel nurses in the NICU with no in-country replacements for these positions could have disastrous outcomes for the patients, staff, and Army in the European command. She called Mr L and Colonel T to advise them of her refusal to follow these orders. She told them that the NICU nurses would not be leaving Germany until acceptable replacements had been processed from the U.S. and had arrived in Germany. Both the Medical Center Commander and the Civilian Personnel Officer protested and advised Colonel A that she was disobeying orders. In the subsequent month, Colonel A consulted with the Chief of the European Command who supported her decision and actions.

DATA COLLECTION AND ASSESSMENT

I. Data Collection and Assessment
   A. Situational Considerations
      1. What situational factors contribute to the ethical dilemma or issue?

   2. How do these situational factors contribute to the ethical dilemma or issue?
B. Health Team Considerations
   1. What persons are most involved in the situation?
   2. What are the relevant backgrounds (e.g., educational level, value orientations) of the persons most involved?
   3. What persons are most affected by the outcome of the decision?
C. Organizational Considerations
   1. What is the nature and mission of the organization
   2. What are the organization's values, policies, and procedures relevant to the situation?

Situational Considerations

The situational factors contributing to the ethical dilemma confronting Colonel A are as follows:

1. *The Army Medical Center provides the only neonatal intensive care services in the European command.* The NICU is the sole neonatal unit in the European command, serving all branches of the military. With the cuts in the budget, civilian personnel stationed at the Army Medical Center for more than five years would be reassigned to the United States within the next sixty days, including more than two thirds of the NICU staff. The ethical issue raised in this situation is: What is the moral responsibility of the Army Medical Department to insure the availability of safe NICU services that meet minimum standards of quality nursing care due to the soldiers and their families? More specifically, despite its scarce resources, isn't the Army morally obliged to take care of its own and to carry out personnel changes that will not compromise standards of nursing care?

2. *Adherence to the military orders to remove experienced nurses from the NICU would endanger the patients.* The implementation of this directive would create a potentially harmful situation for patients, family, and staff in the NICU, one in which high-risk neonates would be receiving care on an understaffed unit or from unskilled nurses. The ethical question arising from this situation is: What is the Army's duty not to inflict harm that could result from the implementation of this directive? In other words, how can safe NICU care be provided with adherence to military orders?

Health Team Considerations

Persons most involved in this situation included Colonel A, the Director of Nursing at the Army Medical Center; Mr L, the Civilian Personnel Officer; Colonel T, the Medical Center Commander; and the neonates and their military families. Other persons involved included the civilian nursing personnel, the staff at the Army Medical Center, and the Chief of the European Command.

Among the persons most involved in the situation, relevant background information included:

1. *Colonel A*—Colonel A had been the Director of Nursing at the Army Medical Center for two years. In this capacity she was very familiar with the personnel needs and management demands of this nursing service. The responsibilities inherent in her position included directing staffing patterns among all the nursing units. Colonel A reported directly to the Commander of the Army Medical Center, and she was responsible for working in a line relationship with the other chiefs within the Army Medical Center.

   Colonel A has a MS in Medical–Surgical Nursing with extensive military education in administration and management. She had been in command of nursing service in two previous assignments and was highly experienced in administrative functions. As an articulate and well-organized nurse administrator, Colonel A had steadily moved up the Army career ladder. She was morally committed to the provision of excellent nursing care within the Center. As the spokesperson for nursing within the Army Medical Center and the European Command, Colonel A frequently found herself representing the health care rights of patients and their families in an effort to safeguard their care.

2. *Mr L*—Mr L was relatively new in his support position as Civilian Personnel Officer for the Army Medical Command, having only been in the position for three months. He was reassigned to this position following the budget cuts at the Department of Defense. He had a reputation among his colleagues for his strong administrative skills and his ability to implement difficult policies with civilian personnel. Despite his unfamiliarity with the needs of the Medical Command, Mr L was convinced of the need to reassign all civilians who had been overseas for more than five years. This conviction was based on his knowledge of the budget deficit and his experience with organizational management.

Mr L had a master's degree in personnel management and had been a career officer for 28 years. Mr L believed in following the letter of the law and abiding by the rules. As a result, he was perceived by his fellow officers as being unwilling to negotiate in work-related matters and as being complicit with authority without regard for the larger human issues.

3. *Colonel T*—Colonel T is a surgeon who had been assigned as Commander to the Army Medical Center during the past six months following his promotion to the rank of colonel. This assignment was his first Medical Center Command, and he was eager to do a good job in his new position. He had not been personally involved with the NICU. While he knew the unit was staffed by several fully qualified neonatology physicians, he was not fully aware of the need for experienced nurses to provide 24-hour care in the NICU.

In his role as Medical Center Commander, Colonel T was still somewhat unsure of his authority, particularly as it related to interdisciplinary issues. For that reason, he was hesitant to overrule the Civilian Personnel Officer regarding the implementation of this policy. In addition, Colonel T was particularly sensitive to criticism from officers in staff line relationships and concerned about his long-term career aspirations in the Army.

4. *Neonates and their families*—The patients were the potential innocent victims in this situation. Clearly the acuity level of the neonates on the NICU ranged from moderate to severe, warranting the need for qualified staff. Moreover, these patients were at high risk for being endangered without specialized nursing care. Despite the seriousness of this situation, the families of the neonates had virtually no knowledge of the decision to remove the qualified civilian nursing personnel from the NICU.

Other persons involved in this situation included the civilian personnel and army nurses who staffed the NICU. These nurses had worked as a team for approximately five years. Through careful and deliberate plans, they had developed the reputation of the NICU as a family-oriented center with technically competent and humanistic care. By removing more than two-thirds of the highly experienced NICU civilian personnel nursing staff over a 60-day period, a void would be created in the unit that would require total reorganization of the nursing personnel in the Medical Center and perhaps elimination of the NICU unit. Replacement of these civilians with newly hired civilian nurses and Army nurses with competencies in neonatology was highly unlikely. Moreover, the highly technical training of the neonatal staff had taken place gradually on the unit during the past five years. It was clear that removal of these civilian nurses in a brief time period would severely compromise the provision of care.

The persons most directly affected by the outcome of this decision were the neonates and their families. In addition, the civilian personnel nurses and the Army staff nurses were affected by the decision. For the civilian personnel nurses the outcome of this decision was time bound, since their reassignment was to be made within a 60-day period. For the Army nurses, the reassignment had the ability to drastically alter their work environment, creating a highly stressful atmosphere and inadequate staffing patterns. The two colonels were also affected by the outcome of this decision, as was the Civilian Personnel Officer. Colonel A was affected because her ability to provide nursing care on the unit was threatened; Colonel T was affected because of his lack of confidence as Medical Commander, which prevented him from questioning these orders; and Mr L was affected because his ability to follow and carry out orders was put to the question.

Organizational Considerations

The mission of the Army Medical Center was to provide health care to military personnel and their families in Western Europe. The goal of the NICU was to provide highly technical, specialized care to neonates born to soldiers and their families in the European Command. Since the NICU services were both needed and deserved by these families, the health care administrators and providers had a responsibility to safeguard this right to health care and to ensure a standard of care for the neonates and their families.

Another factor that must be considered is the organizational culture of the Army. Within the military context, the basic rules of the hierarchy (i.e., group actions) often make it difficult for an individual to act as an independent moral agent.

PROBLEM IDENTIFICATION

II. Problem Identification
   A. Ethical Considerations
      1. What are the ethical considerations related to the case?
      2. Which of these ethical considerations take priority?

B. Nonethical Considerations
1. What are nonethical considerations related to the case (e.g., medical, legal, or factual considerations)?
2. How do the nonethical considerations relate to the ethical considerations?

Ethical Considerations

The major ethical considerations in this case are as follows:

1. *In regard to Colonel A*—How can Colonel A assure that the NICU patients are rendered the health care services they are due, despite the directive limiting the number of qualified nurses to provide this service?
2. *In regard to Mr L*—Should Mr L carry out orders relating to the reassignment of civilian personnel overseas for more than five years, even though these orders would compromise neonatal care in the European Command?
3. *In regard to Colonel T*—Should Colonel T, in attempting to follow the orders from a higher command, limit the nursing care provided to the neonates?
4. *In regard to the neonates and their families*—Should the neonates and their families be given less than they deserve because of scarce nursing resources?

From a justice perspective, the ethical consideration that takes precedence in this case is how to assure that NICU patients are rendered the services they are due so that harm does not befall them.

Nonethical Considerations

The major nonethical consideration in this case was the implementation of a new administrative policy in the Department of Defense budget. This new policy was an administrative response within the Armed Forces Command to cut spending and to trim excess spending in all areas. The stimulus had been the legal mandate by Congress to balance the federal budget. Within this national context, the policy-makers were supportive of fair and just distribution of health care services to military personnel and their families, but expected the allocation of these services would be distributed through the curtailed budget. Since civilian personnel were a major expenditure in the Defense budget, this area had been specifically designated to be cut by Congress.

Other nonethical factors included the personal characteristics of the main players in this situation. Colonel A had a strong sense of professional commitment to the military families whom she served, as well as a commitment to serve her country; Mr L operated from a longstanding commitment to serve his country and to protect his position; and Colonel T, unsure of his position due to his lack of administrative experience, was primarily concerned with his image in his new position, along with a desire to serve his country.

CONSIDERATION OF POSSIBLE ACTIONS: UTILITARIAN THINKING

III. Consideration of Possible Actions
   A. Utilitarian Thinking
      1. How is the principle of utility being defined in this case (e.g., happiness, pleasure, health, etc)?
      2. What are viable actions in the case?
      3. What are predicted consequences of the actions for persons affected by the decision?
      4. From the predicted consequences, what is the intrinsic value and disvalue for each viable consequence?
      5. What possible action(s) produce the best consequences overall for happiness, pleasure, health, etc and the least unhappiness, disvalue, displeasure, etc for persons affected, or most affected, by the decision?

Definition of the Principle of Utility

For Colonel A the principle of utility is defined as the greatest good for those most affected by the decision (neonates and their families). The intrinsic value held by Colonel A, then, is rendering quality health care to the neonates and their families who deserve it. In contrast, Mr L and Colonel T essentially are not involved with the principle of utility or utilitarian thinking as their primary focus was following orders and/or preserving career aspirations.

Applying the principle of utility to justice, as was done in this case, has been challenged when consequences become less than maximal. When using the utilitarian perspective, the moral imperative is that one consistently attempts to determine the most favorable action and then pursues that action to maximize valuable consequences. The focus becomes a case of balancing the motives as a means of producing the end result, rather than reaching consensus on the morality of an action (Beauchamp, 1982, p. 98).

Viable Actions

Viable actions for consideration in this case include:

1. Ensure that the neonates and their families receive the care they are due by refusing to send the qualified civilian nurses home until experienced replacements are available.
2. Shut down the NICU temporarily until qualified nursing replacements become available.

The argument for the first viable action (ensuring care) proceeds as follows: The neonates and their families deserve the specialty care offered in the NICU and are in need of the care provided by the nurses in the NICU. It should be noted that this first viable action is a temporary solution in effect until the qualified replacements become available. From a utilitarian perspective of justice, this argument is morally justified because it enables the neonates who are most in need to receive the care they are due. Without such care, harm would come to them. The second viable action (shutting down the unit) might be morally justified according to the utilitarian perspective because it could be argued that this position takes into consideration the consequences for everyone involved, including military personnel.

Predicted Consequences

For the persons most affected by the decision, predicted consequences are as follows:

	Care ensured	Unit shut down
1. *For Colonel A*	• uphold professional ethics and standards of nursing care • uphold Medical Center goals	• neonates and families receive less than they are due • pain of seeing potential patients not receive care

	Care ensured	*Unit shut down*
	• potential reprimand for insubordination	• potential loss of life if unit not available
	• violation of military policy and federal law	• facilitate implementation of military policy and federal law
		• violation of conscience re-garding beneficence
		• violation of nursing code of ethics
2. *For Mr L*	• lack of adherence to the military policy and federal law	• facilitate implementation of military policy and federal law
	• violation of conscience regarding fidelity to others	• uphold military goal
3. *For Colonel T*	• needed care is pro-vided to neonates and families	• uphold military goal
	• long-term career goals jeopardized	• facilitate implementation of military policy and federal law
		• violation of medical code of ethics
		• violation of consience re-garding beneficence
4. *Neonates*	• neonates and families receive care they are due	• specialized care of neo-nates is eliminated

Intrinsic Value/Disvalue of Consequences

The main intrinsic value operating for Colonel A based on the principle of justice, is the provision that the neonates and their families receive the care they are due. On the other hand, the primary intrinsic values operating for Colonel T and Mr L are loyalty to the military system and concern with self if orders are disobeyed.

Outcomes of Actions Regarding Happiness/Unhappiness

According to Colonel A, the greatest good would be served by refusing to send the qualified civilian NICU nurses home until qualified replace-ments arrived. These actions would produce the greatest happiness and freedom from pain for the neonates and their families and for Colonel A. By taking this action, the neonates and their families would receive their just due and have their health care needs met. On the other hand, for Colonel T and Mr L, the greatest happiness would occur if the military policy and federal law were not compromised, even on a temporary basis.

CONSIDERATION OF POSSIBLE ACTIONS: DEONTOLOGICAL THINKING

III. Consideration of Possible Actions, continued
   B. Deontological Thinking
      1. What ethical rules and principles are in conflict?[2]
      2. What duties emerge from these ethical rules and principles?
      3. Which of these duties are in conflict with equal or stronger duties?
      4. If a conflict exists, which duties derived from moral rules and principles produce the greatest balance of rightness over wrongness?

Ethical Rules and Principles in Conflict

The major ethical rules and/or principles in conflict in this case are as follows:

1. *In regard to Colonel A*—The principle of justice in relation to the macroallocation of resources as mandated by Congress is in conflict with the needed microallocation of resources on the NICU.
2. *In regard to Colonel T*—The rule of fidelity to uphold military policy is in conflict with those aspects of the principle of beneficence as it relates to the prevention of harm to the neonates and their families.
3. *In regard to Mr L*—The rule of fidelity to uphold military orders is in conflict with the principle of justice as it relates to the neonates receiving their just due regarding nursing personnel.

---

[2]**Note:** A role utilitarian would also raise questions about ethical rules and principles, but would assess the rules in terms of consequences instead of duties.

Duties Emerging from Rules and Principles

Based on these rules and principles, the following prima facie duties emerge in this case:

1. From the principle of justice emerges the duty to provide the neonates and their families with the care they deserve.
2. From the principle of fidelity emerges the duty to abide by military policy and obey orders.
3. From the principle of beneficence emerges the duty to safeguard the neonates by preventing the potential harm that could result to them if the NICU was closed temporarily.

Duties in Conflict

The prima facie duties in conflict in this case stem from an interplay between the principles of justice and beneficence and the rules of fidelity. Colonel A sought to ensure that high-risk neonates received the care they were due so that they would not be harmed. Colonel T and Mr L both operated from their duty to honor their obligations to the military system.

The burden of the responsibility for the ethical decision making is thrust on Colonel A because both Mr L and Colonel T are unwilling to deviate from orders. They are both prepared to implement the policy by removing the civilian nursing personnel from the NICU, despite the fact that the stronger duty to ensure care overrides the obligation to follow military orders in this case.

Greatest Balance of Rightness Over Wrongness

For Colonel A the moral duty of ensuring that the neonates receive the care they are due overrides her duty to follow orders. Colonel A believed she did not need to obey orders that she thought were immoral. For her, the just distribution of nursing resources to the neonates and their families produced more rightness than adherence to a policy that most likely would have caused the NICU to be closed down until qualified nursing replacements could be assigned to the Army Medical Center.

Since the duty of fidelity overrides justice for Colonel T and Mr L, they are both unwilling to take measures to ensure the neonates and their families get the standard of care they are due.

DECISION AND SELECTION OF COURSE OF ACTION

IV. Decision and Selection of Course of Action
   A. Contribution of Internal/Group Factors
     1. For whom is the decision being made?
     2. Who should decide?
     3. What biases/values of persons involved in the decision affect the decision?
   B. Contribution of External Factors
     1. What institutional factors are affecting the decision and selected course of action?
     2. What legal factors are affecting the decision and selected course of action?
     3. What social factors are affecting the decision and selected course of action?
   C. Quality of Decision and Course of Action
     1. What decision is being made?
     2. What course of action to implement the decision is being made?
     3. In light of the preceding factors, is the decision being made and the course of action to be taken ones that can still be morally justified?
     4. If not, how can the decision being made and the course of action to be taken be altered so that they are morally justified?
     5. Is the selected course of action based on the decision implementable?

Contribution of Internal/Group Factors

The biases and values of the persons involved in this decision played a significant role in the formulation and outcome of the decision. In this case, the decision was being made by the health care administrative group for the neonates and their families. As is often the case, this group was unaware of the ethical dilemma faced by Colonel A as she struggled with this decision. When confronted with the decision, Mr L and Colonel T selected the conservative route, opting to follow orders and protect their own personal interests. Mr L, in his role as Civilian Personnel Officer, was accountable for the reassignment of the civilian nurses in question. He did not have a clear understanding, however, of the seriousness of this situation for the patients, their families, or Colonel A and her staff. Clearly, following orders in this situation relieves the independent agent of his responsibility for moral decision making, which cannot be morally justified in this case. Neither Mr L nor Colonel T sought to understand the motives and/or values driving Colonel A's decision at the time.

Although Colonel T understood more than Mr L the implications of shutting down the NICU, he was unwilling to risk his reputation or long-term career aspirations to ensure that justice was served for the neonates. Rather, he followed the orders and allowed Colonel A to assume the leadership role in this case. Colonel A stood her moral ground as she perceived it and sought to protect the health care rights of the neonates and their families. Had Colonel A not exercised the strength of her convictions and refused to follow these orders, it is possible that the NICU might have remained open without adequate staff or closed temporarily. Both of these plans would have severely compromised the care of neonates and potentially endangered the lives of newborns in the European Command. Because of Mr L's inability to choose the most justifiable course of action, Colonel A was morally obligated to act to safeguard the rights of the neonates needing health care.

The values of the individuals involved in this case affected the decision selected. Colonel A's decision was based on her belief that nurses have a duty to ensure patients' rights to health care through the allocation of nursing care. Due to his lack of self-confidence and inexperience in the position, Colonel T's values were less clear, although they stemmed from his fear of jeopardizing his position. Mr L's values culminated from his previous military experiences with problems that he perceived as having much more serious consequences, such as a formal reprimand for not implementing policy for which he was accountable.

Contribution of External Factors

Several external factors were noted in this case. The most salient institutional factor contributing to the ethical dilemma was the new administrative policy curtailing the length of overseas assignments for civilian personnel. Both Mr L and Colonel T were affected by the organizational culture of the military in that the obeying of military orders is highly valued.

Federal policy also affected this case. As was discussed earlier, the rationale for curtailing the Defense budget originated with the attempts of the United States Congress to balance the federal budget deficit. Hence, the new policy for overseas civilian personnel was an attempt by the Army to reduce costs, with many of the specific procedures for implementing this policy left unresolved.

Social factors played an interesting part in this case. All the potential decision makers were of similar rank and/or staff position. The line of authority regarding the final decisions in the Army Medical Center rested with Colonel T by virtue of his position as Medical Center Commander; however, because Colonel T was uncertain of his moral obligations in this situation and refused to question orders, Colonel A felt morally obligated to refuse to follow orders for the protection of the welfare of the neonates and their families.

Quality of Decision and Course of Action

Colonel A's decision (refusing to allow the civilian neonatal nurses to leave until military nurses became available) enabled the neonates and their families to get the care they were due. Thus justice was served for the neonates in this case. The course of action selected by Colonel A was eventually supported by the Chief of the Army Medical Command in Europe; however, the initial lack of support she received from Mr L and Colonel T created a difficult administrative and moral situation for Colonel A.

Colonel A sought to provide the neonates and their families with the care they deserved. This course of action was morally justified according to the principles of justice and beneficence because the infants received the care they deserved and were protected from harm in the process. The morally relevant properties of the right to health care and the need for health care were considered as the basis for distributing nursing care in this case.

REFLECTION ON DECISION
AND COURSE OF ACTION

V. Reflection on Decision and Course of Action
    A. Reflection on Decision
        1. Was the decision that was made the one that was actually acted upon? If not, why not?

2. Did the decision that was made accomplish its intended purpose? If not, why not?
3. In retrospect, do you believe the decision that was made was morally good or right? Why? Why not?
B. Reflection on Course of Action
1. Was the selected course of action carried out in the manner intended? Why? Why not?
2. Did the selected course of action accomplish its intended purpose? If not, why not?
3. In retrospect, do you believe the course of action taken was morally right or good? If not, why not?

Colonel A went against a military command and acted on her decision to distribute nursing care on the NICU, despite a move to implement a new order which could severely curtail nursing care in the NICU. Her decision accomplished its intended purpose of providing nursing care to the neonates and their families until experienced NICU nurses became available (about six months after the initial memo). This decision was morally good because the neonates received the care they needed and deserved. The decision also protected the infants from the potential harm of an inadequately staffed or closed NICU.

The selected course of action was carried out, and this action accomplished its intended purpose of distributing scarce nursing resources to those due the services and in need of health care. From a utilitarian perspective, the selected course of action resulted in the greatest good for those most affected by the decision because the neonates and their families received the care they needed, even though the cost reduction policies were delayed.

From a deontological perspective, the moral duty to distribute this care outweighed the moral duty to obey orders for the implementation of the cost reduction policy.

CASE COMMENTARY[3]

I experienced many feelings as I struggled with the case of justice for the neonates. I was particularly concerned that the neonates receive the nursing

---

[3]Case Commentary by: **Brigadier General Clara Adams-Ender, RN, MS, MMAS,** Chief, United States Army Nurse Corps, Washington, D.C.

care they were due. I remember thinking that the neonates were helpless to care for themselves and that my two hands would certainly not be enough alone. I felt anger and frustration with Mr L because he seemed to be more concerned with obeying the rules and conforming to policy without regard for jeopardizing the lives of the neonates. Moreover, Colonel T's response was equally frustrating because he knew both sides of the issue and refused to make a decision, even after the factual data were presented. In my opinion, his indecision still represented a decision which mitigated against the neonates.

The preceding analysis was most enlightening for me because it provided an opportunity to become more familiar with the analytical process one could use in ethical decision making. In retrospect, perhaps I did not give enough credence and consideration to Mr L's point of view. After having read the analysis and the application of the principle of justice, I concluded that I would have arrived at the same conclusion but would have been more aware of how I got to that point.

The outcome of this case has demonstrated that justice is part of a consistent pattern in my style of decision making in executive nursing management. I value justice highly in administrative decisions. As a nurse executive I have many opportunities to make decisions about scarce resource distribution. In all instances, the principle of justice is weighed not only for the patients involved but also for the staff and the military organization as a whole. When prioritizing decision making about scarce resources, I still tend to give the greatest consideration to the needs of patients. I have pondered my rationale for doing this and have concluded that the incurrence of public trust as a licensed professional necessitates that I accurately represent their interests in any negotiations about their nursing care since they are unable to do so themselves. In that sense, I must be the patient advocate and ensure that those interests are clearly articulated and given serious consideration.

Summary. This case provides the reader with a perspective on the principle of justice as it relates to the allocation of scarce nursing resources. The ethical principles of justice and beneficence and the duty of fidelity are explored in the context of the military system. The decision and course of action are analyzed according to the utilitarian and deontological approaches, and are commented upon by the nurse administrator who faced the dilemma.

| CASE STUDY 2 |

The Inappropriate Distribution
of Primary Health Care Funds[4]

The Division of Primary Care in the State Health Department funded primary care, home health, health promotion, and disease prevention services throughout the state. Several sources of state funding existed for the Division of Primary Care, as well as federal funds allocated by the United States Department of Health and Human Services for designated programs. These federal funds were specifically earmarked for disease prevention in the area of pediatric services.

As the Director of the Division of Primary Care, Ms M, a nurse, held one of the highest level positions in the State Health Department in a rural Mid-Atlantic state. Although a nurse, Ms M's position was not administered by nursing; instead, she reported directly to the Director of the State Health Department. Within the Division of Primary Care, Ms M was responsible for monitoring the distribution of several million dollars of state and federal appropriations and supervising the programs funded through her division. A 31-year-old nurse with a master's degree in public health, Ms M had been employed in this position for less than two months. Her predecessor had been an elderly physician who had health problems and experienced difficulty in managing the administrative demands of the position during his 35-year tenure. He had particular problems in complying with the federal regulations related to the distribution of federal funds.

Ms M had received regular requests for state and federal funds from Agency X that served a large, poor district (District X) in the state. Agency X combined health department, home health, and primary care services for the indigent population of District X. The indigent population of District X consisted primarily of two subgroups: elderly persons with chronic illnesses and young families with infants and small children. In the past three years, the Pediatric Program funded by the federal government had been poorly administered by the staff of Agency X. No formal evaluation of this problem had been conducted by Ms M's predecessor. These poor administrative practices had, in turn, limited the types of pediatric services available to families with young children in District X. These activities had been attributed to error and a lack of understanding of the federal policy in the Health Department. Specifically, it was alleged that federal funds appropriated for the delivery of pediatric services

---

[4]Case Submitted by: Janet L. Chapin, RN, MPH, Administrator, Underserved Women, American College of Obstetricians and Gynecologists, Washington, D.C.

to children and families had been used to supplement funding for the home care program for elderly persons in District X.

The Director of Agency X was a physician in his 50s who had been in the position for 20 years. He was well known for his ability to identify primary care needs and to secure funding for these programs at the national, state, and local levels. Dr X frequently reminded Ms M of his long-term influence and power in the state and District X. During these interactions, Dr X would allude to her limited experiences as an administrator in the Health Department.

Ms M knew the statistics reported by Dr X and his staff in relation to pediatric services seemed implausible. According to the data reported by Agency X, few physical exams were being performed, yet excess money remained in the budget toward the end of each fiscal year. The money that would have been used to perform these exams was being used to supplement the home care program for the elderly. Whenever Ms M questioned him about these inconsistencies, Dr X cited his overriding concerns were the needy pediatric and elderly groups in the community and the lack of staff for collecting and summarizing the data for the Pediatric Program. He also made several references to Ms M's lack of longevity in her position.

Ms M had not conducted a formal review and/or evaluation of Dr X in the short time she had been there. She wished to avoid an adversarial relationship with Dr X and therefore avoided confronting him directly on this matter. She reported these concerns to the Director of the Health Department, who reminded Ms M that she was accountable for assuring that the Pediatric Program operate in compliance with the federal regulations, despite Dr X's poor administrative skills.

Ms M was deeply aware that Agency X was the sole provider of pediatric services for the indigent children. Knowing no other organizations could provide a similar service in District X and knowing both populations needed the care left her in a quandary. Yet, she did not have the human or material resources to provide services to both the indigent children and the homebound elderly. Since federal funds were allocated specifically for the pediatric health care services, Ms M felt morally and legally obligated to assure that the indigent children in District X received the care they were due from the Pediatric Program.

The strategy Ms M developed was to institute several new policies for the distribution of funds. The policies became requirements for all agencies in the state to receive funds from the Division of Primary Care. First, the policy for the distribution of funds for the Pediatric Program was contingent on documenting and submitting monthly reports about program performance according to a specified format. Second, peer administrators from the 20 districts in the State Health Department were assigned to make periodic unannounced site visits to all agencies funded by the Division of Primary Care. Finally, Ms M convened a task force with the charge of developing procedures for these policies and reviewing these reports at monthly intervals. Members of the Task Force included agency administrators of all the state-funded primary care programs and representatives from the federal government. Through these policies, she created a safety net whereby Dr X, should he continue not to follow administrative procedures, would receive reprimands and potentially lose his job.

With these administrative measures in place, Dr X and his staff did submit monthly reports. In conjunction with these monthly reports, peer administrators were assigned to Agency X to assist Dr X and his staff in the interpretation of these policies and procedures. During the course of these site visits, the peer administrators found and corrected several misinterpretations concerning documentation and the conduct of the Pediatric Program at Agency X. These errors were corrected at Agency X with the follow-up by the site visitors and the subsequent review by the Task Force. Through these new administrative measures, Dr X and his staff improved the delivery of care in the Pediatric Program, followed guidelines for the distribution of monies, and sought new funding to support home care programs for the elderly.

DATA COLLECTION AND ASSESSMENT

I. Data Collection and Assessment
    A. Situational Considerations
        1. What situational factors contribute to the ethical dilemma or issue?
        2. How do these situational factors contribute to the ethical dilemma or issue?
    B. Health Team Considerations
        1. What persons are most involved in the situation?
        2. What are the relevant backgrounds (e.g., educational level, value orientations) of the persons most involved?
        3. What persons are most affected by the outcome of the decision?
    C. Organizational Considerations
        1. What is the nature and mission of the organization?
        2. What are the organization's values, policies, and procedures relevant to the situation?

Situational Considerations

The situational factors contributing to the ethical dilemma and the ways they contributed are identified as follows:

1. *Federal funds had been allocated to the states to subsidize pediatric primary care programs.* Federal funds had been granted to supplement the delivery of pediatric services because of the significant number of low-income families in the population unable to provide primary care for their children. These funds had been earmarked for children because a decision had been made by public policy makers that the health of the nation's children was a higher priority than that of other special population groups, such as the elderly and chronically ill. The ethical issue is: On what moral basis can the distribution of these funds to the children be justified when the elderly homebound have health care needs equivalent to those of the indigent children?

2. *Unspent federal funds had been used to supplement a home care program for the elderly, rather than to improve pediatric primary care services in District X.* Despite the fact that these funds were specifically designated by the federal government for the Pediatric Program, Dr X had allowed the unspent funds to be used to support the home care program for the elderly. Dr X was faced with a conflict about how to deliver health care services to two groups in equal need; these groups consisted of mothers and their babies, and elderly families with multiple chronic illnesses. Each of these two subgroups had definite health care needs; however, monies had only been allocated by the federal government for the delivery of pediatric health care services, so the children were meant to be the designated recipients of these funds. Based on this situation the following ethical issue can be raised: On what moral basis did Dr X provide health care services to both the indigent children and the elderly persons in District X? Specifically, what are the morally relevant properties on which these funds were distributed? What are the morally relevant properties on which these funds should be distributed in the future?

3. *Ms M feared that the children in District X would not receive the primary care services they were due.* As the relatively new Director of the Primary Care Division, Ms M had spoke with Dr X without success regarding inconsistencies in program spending. In each of these interactions, Dr X had alluded to the possibility of Ms M losing her job should she pursue these inconsistencies. If

she lost her position or was forced to make formal accusations against Dr X, Ms M risked the possibility of the federal government funds not being distributed to District X. This could result in harm for the children who could potentially lose pediatric services if these funds were withdrawn. The ethical issue in this situation is: How to assure the continued distribution of funds for the Pediatric Program in District X and assure the children received the care to which they were entitled? In particular, what moral values must guide Ms M's administrative actions to assure the distribution of funds to the Pediatric Program in District X?

Health Team Considerations

Persons most involved in this situation included Ms M, who was Director of the Primary Care Division in the State Department of Health; Dr X, who was Director of Agency X; and the indigent children in District X. Other persons involved included the state and federal agency administrators, the Chief of the State Health Department, and the homebound elderly.

Among the persons most involved in the situation, relevant background information included:

1. *Ms M*—As the Director of the Primary Care Division, Ms M held a high administrative position within the Department of Health. Her position responsibilities entailed the oversight of several health programs and the distribution of several million dollars of state and federal funds. Ms M's specific administrative duties encompassed management of a wide variety of health professionals, including physicians, health care administrators, nurses, pharmacists, social workers, and physical therapists. She reported directly to the Chief of the State Health Department. Due to her relative inexperience in this job, Ms M was particularly sensitive to potential criticism from her supervisors and colleagues.

   Ms M was a 31-year-old nurse administrator with a master's degree in public health. She was an effective, intelligent administrator who had been in this position less than two months and had long-term aspirations for career advancement in health care administration. Despite the interdisciplinary nature of her position, Ms M's values stemmed from her nursing roots. First and foremost, she felt a moral obligation to distribute the federal and state funds for health resources to the needy communities in her state. She also had a legal obligation to distribute these funds according to the federal and state policies governing these funds.

2. *Dr X*—The Director of Agency X was a physician in his 50s who had worked in this position for the past 20 years. Dr X was well known for his ability to acquire state and federal funding for his programs and his ability to identify health care needs within the community. His ability to implement and manage these programs had not been questioned by the previous Director of Primary Care because they were friends. Dr X's major fault was that he did not pay attention to details about the policies and procedures for using state and federal funds; instead he considered this "red tape a waste of time." Dr X felt a conflict about the allocation of funds solely to the Pediatric Program, for he believed the elderly homebound in District X were also deserving of care. He cited a lack of staff and resources in his agency to provide care to both of these indigent groups and to analyze the data needed by the Health Department. To further complicate the situation, Dr X was a close personal friend of the Chief of the Health Department. They had worked well together to establish the policy and funding base for primary health care in the state. Administratively, Dr X answered to the Chief of the Health Department for medical matters and to the Director of the Primary Care Division for programmatic matters.

3. *Indigent children in District X*—The infants and small children in need lived in a large, rural district in the state. The indigent children were members of young, relatively uneducated families. The majority of this group worked as laborers or farmers, and their income was contingent on the economic and general welfare of the state. Since these families fell into the low-income bracket, the children were eligible for free primary care screening, physicals, and preventive follow-up. Without this federal program, these children would not receive the care they needed because their families could not afford it.

4. *Indigent, homebound elderly in District X*—A significant aging population lived in District X. These elderly individuals had multiple chronic diseases and lived primarily at home due to a limited number of life care resources in the district. Since the majority of these individuals were lifetime residents who were supported by their families, their primary care and home care needs were highly visible in the community. Their needs for

home care services were legitimate, yet the majority of these services were not reimburseable through Medicare or Medicaid. The policy decisions related to home care for the sick elderly were the subject of long-term debate at the federal level, but, as yet, no consensus has been achieved by policy makers. Although policy makers felt a moral obligation to provide a decent minimum standard of health care for the elderly, controversy existed about how to define and distribute that health care.

The persons most affected by the outcome of this decision were the indigent children of District X, since they had no other resources for pediatric coverage. If the funds were used solely for the children in the Pediatric Program, the elderly homebound would lose services. On the other hand, if the funds were used to support both the Pediatric Program and the home care program for the elderly, the indigent children could lose the health care services to which they were entitled. Both Ms M and Dr X also were affected by the outcome of this decision. Ms M was affected because she was ultimately responsible for the distribution of funds for the implementation of these programs; she was in a position to rectify this situation because the funds had a legal designation. Therefore Ms M felt morally and legally obliged to distribute funds as they were intended for the indigent children in District X. Of secondary note, Ms M felt her job would be jeopardized if she openly challenged Dr X about the type of service provided by federal funds. Likewise, she felt her job would be in jeopardy if she allowed the extra funds to be used in support of the elderly homecare program. Either situation had the potential to preclude pediatric services from the children in need of them. Dr X was affected insofar as his personal and professional integrity and his job security were under scrutiny and open to question.

Organizational Considerations

The goal of the Division of Primary Care of the State Health Department was to oversee and fund several programs delivering primary care services to special populations in need of health care across the state. The goal of Agency X was to provide primary care services to the persons unable to afford private health care services in their district. Directed by these organizational goals, the providers and health care administrators have a responsibility to assure that individuals due services receive those services. The problem in this case resulted because the pediatric services for the children in District X were not being received.

PROBLEM IDENTIFICATION

II. Problem Identification
  A. Ethical Considerations
    1. What are ethical considerations related to the case?
    2. Which of these ethical considerations take priority?
  B. Nonethical Considerations
    1. What are nonethical considerations related to the case (e.g., medical, legal, or factual considerations)?
    2. How do the nonethical considerations relate to the ethical considerations?

Ethical Considerations

The major ethical considerations in this case are as follows:

1. *In regard to the needy indigent groups in District X*—How can the needs of both groups be met when the funds have been designated solely for the children by the federal government?
2. *In regard to Ms M*—How can Ms M assure that the children in District X receive the Pediatric Services to which they are entitled without losing her job and causing further harm to these children?
3. *In regard to Dr X*—How can Dr X meet the needs of the children and elderly in District X when money is allocated only for the children?

The ethical consideration that takes priority in this situation is whether the children in District X should receive the services to which they were entitled.

Nonethical Considerations

Several nonethical considerations need to be analyzed in this case. First and foremost is the lack of accountability regarding policy and procedures for the spending of federal funds. Administrative measures had not been taken to limit these inconsistencies prior to Ms M's attempts to deal with this situation. The practice, prior to Ms M's tenure, had been to ignore the errors made by Dr X and his staff. The illegality of ignoring noncompliance with federal policy and funding criteria is a primary concern in this case. Yet, the decisions leading to the formulation of health policy (law) to allocate funds only for the children in this case created ethical conflicts for Dr X and Ms M. Another nonethical factor was Dr X's longstanding friendship with the Chief of the Health Department and Ms M's relative inexperience in her position as Director of the Division of Primary Care. Such factors made Ms M afraid that if she dealt directly with Dr X on the funding issues, she could lose her job, eliminating the distribution of funds to the children who needed them.

CONSIDERATION OF POSSIBLE ACTIONS: UTILITARIAN THINKING

III. Consideration of Possible Actions
   A. Utilitarian Thinking
      1. How is the principle of utility being defined in this case (e.g., happiness, pleasure, health, etc)?
      2. What are viable actions in the case?
      3. What are predicted consequences of the actions for persons affected by the decision?
      4. From the predicted consequences, what is the intrinsic value and disvalue for each viable consequence?
      5. What possible action(s) produce the best consequences overall for happiness, pleasure, health, etc and the least unhappiness, disvalue, displeasure, etc for persons affected, or most affected, by the decision?

Definition of the Principle of Utility

The principle of utility, as described in Chapter 2, holds that pleasure and freedom from pain are the *only* desirable ends. As such, all desirable things are a means to the promotion of pleasure and the prevention of pain (Mill, 1861/1979, p. 7). In this particular case, pleasure can be associated with the provision of health care, and pain can be associated with the lack of health care for the indigent children in District X.

Likewise, the principle of utility is based on the premise that the rightness of an act is determined in part by the intrinsic value of its consequences and the effect of these consequences on all those affected by the act (Mill, 1861/1979, p. 16). Since justice, by definition, implies that actions are fair and/or equal, Ms M's primary concern is to assure that funds are distributed fairly and equitably to provide health care for the children, since the children are entitled to the primary care services by law. Although the elderly have legitimate needs for health care also, the monies were allocated at the federal level for the primary care of the children.

Viable Actions

From a utilitarian perspective, the following viable actions can be considered in this case:

1. Allow the funds to be distributed to Agency X for the Pediatric Program with a plan for assuring the fair and equitable distribution of all allocated funds to the children in need.
2. Confront Dr X regarding the spending of federal monies to supplement the home care program for the elderly.

The argument for the first viable action (distributing all the allocated funds to the Pediatric Program with a plan) is that the children are entitled to have these services according to federal law. Therefore, the funds for the Pediatric Program rightfully belong to the children and should be used to meet their health care needs. By developing a system for distribution of these monies, Ms M could be relatively certain that the children would get what they deserved. The second viable action (confronting Dr X) is justified because Dr X's funding of both programs for the past three years had been a reflection of his moral dilemma concerning the needs of the elderly and pediatric indigent populations in District X. His actions had restricted the types of services the children had received. Thus it could be argued that unless Dr X is confronted with these actions, he will continue to abuse the rights of the indigent children, delaying a valid request to the Director of the Health Department for services for the elderly.

Predicted Consequences

The predicted consequences are listed for the individuals or groups most affected by the decision:

	Monies distributed to Pediatric Program with plan	Dr X confronted
1. *For Ms M*	• potential for children to receive care they deserve • development of procedures to monitor distribution of funds • children's health care needs are potentially met • uphold administrative goals • possible administrative pressure due to implementation of new program • lack of health care for homebound elderly	• children receive care they deserve • potential to communicate pressing needs of the elderly to Director of Health Department • children's health care needs may not be met because Ms M loses job and program is withdrawn • potential loss of job • stress associated with confronting Dr X • potential lack of health care for homebound elderly
2. *For children*	• potentially receive the care they are due • health care needs may be met	• right to health care services may be respected • children may not get what they are due
3. *For Dr X*	• potential for children to receive health care they are due • pain of administrative surveillance • potential for lobbying for home care services for elderly	• program may be discontinued because of failure to comply with policy • pain of possible loss of job • loss of personal and professional integrity • mental anguish

Intrinsic Value/Disvalue of Consequences

The primary goal for Ms M, from a justice perspective, is that the funds owed the children from the Pediatric Program are distributed for their designated purpose. Inherent in this goal is the intrinsic value of helping the indigent children get their health care needs met. Concurrently, the elderly will probably lose home care services. On the other hand, from a justice-as-fairness perspective, direct confrontation of Dr X regarding his spending actions in Agency X may result in a lack of services for both the children and the elderly, ultimately placing Ms M's and Dr X's jobs in jeopardy.

Outcomes of Actions Regarding Happiness/Unhappiness

According to a utilitarian approach, the greatest good for the greatest number would be served by developing a system to monitor the distribution of funds to the indigent children. The consequences of this action would produce the greatest happiness by providing pediatric services to those who deserve them, and, in particular, to those most affected by them. For Ms M, this means she would meet her obligation to provide health care to the indigent children and would not risk losing her job. The indigent children would receive their just due and have their health care needs met. Dr X would receive the administrative supervision he needed and would be forced to comply with the policies of the Pediatric Program. Therefore justice would be served and disruption of the entire system avoided. Although the indigent elderly could potentially lose benefits under this plan, they were not due these services from a distributive justice perspective. Using this approach, justice would be served for the elderly if they could have their needs communicated to the appropriate decision makers.

CONSIDERATION OF POSSIBLE ACTIONS: DEONTOLOGICAL THINKING

III. Consideration of Possible Actions, continued
   B. Deontological Thinking
      1. What ethical rules and principles are in conflict?[5]
      2. What duties emerge from these ethical rules and principles?
      3. Which of these duties are in conflict with equal or stronger duties?
      4. If a conflict exists, which duties derived from moral rules and principles produce the greatest balance of rightness over wrongness?

---

[5]**Note:** A role utilitarian would also raise questions about ethical rules and principles but would assess the rules in terms of consequences instead of duties.

Ethical Rules and Principles in Conflict

Major ethical rules and/or principles in conflict are presented as they relate to the decision makers in this case. They are as follows:

1. *In regard to Ms M*—The principle of nonmaleficence (i.e., Ms M's desire to do no harm to the indigent children in District X) is in conflict with the principle of justice that focuses on the allocation of health resources (i.e., the delivery of pediatric services).
2. *In regard to Dr X*—The principle of beneficence (e.g., the duty to do good) is in conflict with the principle of respect for quality of life (i.e., for children in the Pediatric Program and elderly in the home care program), as well as the principle of justice as fairness.

Duties Emerging from Rules and Principles

Based on these rules and principles, the following prima facie duties are identified:

1. From the principle of justice emerges the duty to insure that the children get the health care they are due.
2. From the principle of beneficence emerges the duty to safeguard the health care of the children by implementing accountability measures to improve the care due to the children.
3. From the principle of nonmaleficence emerges the duty to do no harm to the children or the elderly, that is, to make certain that the children receive the services they are due from the Pediatric Program and to assure the needs of the elderly are communicated to the appropriate state authorities.
4. From the principle of respect for quality of life emerges the duty to promote the health needs of those in need, that is, the indigent children and elderly.

Duties in Conflict

Dr X resolved his conflict by using the unspent funds in the Pediatric Program to supplement the home care program for the elderly. The burden of decision making rests with Ms M, since dealing directly with Dr X about this problem has the potential to stop funding for the program and to produce serious outcomes for her and Dr X. Therefore, a prima facie duty conflict emerges for Ms M:

The conflict between the duty to distribute the funds for the Pediatric Program with a plan to assure the children receive the care they are due and the duty to do no harm to the children and/or the elderly.

Ms M is the primary decision maker in this case because she is accountable for all administrative matters related to the Division of Primary Care, and Dr X has refused to take an active role in resolving this issue. The indigent children and the elderly are unaware of the conflict.

Greatest Balance of Rightness Over Wrongness

For Ms M, the moral duty of distributing funds for the Pediatric Program with a plan for systematically monitoring the Program was more justifiable than confronting Dr X and potentially alerting the federal authorities about Dr X's use of the funds. When Ms M's motives are considered in conjunction with the moral standards of these acts, the obligation to deliver the services to the children outweighs the obligation to report Dr X's use of the funds. With Ms M's plan for evaluation and budget accountability for Dr X in distributing funds for pediatric services, her motives are morally justified.

DECISION AND SELECTION OF COURSE OF ACTION

IV. Decision and Selection of Course of Action
   A. Contribution of Internal/Group Factors
      1. For whom is the decision being made?
      2. Who should decide?
      3. What biases/values of persons involved in the situation affect the decision?
   B. Contribution of External Factors
      1. What institutional factors are affecting the decision and selected course of action?
      2. What legal factors are affecting the decision and selected course of action?
      3. What social factors are affecting the decision and the selected course of action?

C. Quality of Decision and Course of Action
1. What decision is being made?
2. What course of action to implement the decision is being made?
3. In light of the preceding factors, is the decision being made and the course of action to be taken ones that can still be morally justified?
4. If not, how can the decision being made and the course of action to be taken be altered so that they are morally justified?
5. Is the selected course of action based on the decision implementable?

Contribution of Internal/Group Factors

Formulating the decision and enacting its course is dependent on the biases and values of the persons involved in the decision-making process. The primary group for whom this decision is made is the indigent children in District X. According to the facts of this case, this group is unaware that an ethical dilemma is affecting their health care. Likewise, a decision is being made for Dr X, who has not conformed to the federal policies and standards designated by the Division of Primary Care. As Director of the Division of Primary Care, Ms M is the decision maker in this case. Since funds were distributed to Agency X via the Division, Ms M is accountable for the spending patterns and the care provided by Dr X and his staff. Although the question of who should decide seems apparent in this case, Dr X also has several decisions to make. As noted, he did not comply with administrative policies pertaining to the distribution of funds. This refusal affected the indigent children and elderly groups in District X as well as Ms M. Had he complied with federal regulations, he could have maintained control over the decision-making process; however, because Dr X did not comply, Ms M was obligated to act to safeguard the rights of the indigent children in need of health care.

The values of Ms M and Dr X affected the decision selected. Ms M's primary decision stemmed from her belief that the children needed and deserved the health care due them. Dr X's decision, on the other hand, stemmed from his belief that both the children and the elderly needed health care. His belief, however, led to noncompliance with federal policies and standards.

Ms M's decision to institute new policies and procedures made the distribution of funds contingent on adhering to administrative procedures and submitting required data at monthly intervals. With this decision, she was able to provide the indigent children in District X with the care they were due and to comply with federal regulations for the Pediatric Program. Likewise, Dr X's actions were monitored monthly by herself and his peers. This action provided the data needed to specifically evaluate his performance and compliance with policy and procedures.

Contribution of External Factors

Several external factors were noted in this case. The most significant institutional factor affecting the decision-making process was the lack of administrative measures in the Division of Primary Care and Agency X to assure funds were used to deliver health services for which they were designated. With the failure of Agency X to adhere to federal regulations, Ms M was ultimately responsible for the ways in which funds were used.

Legal issues were threaded throughout this case. Since federal policies had not been followed during the years prior to Ms M's administrative tenure, she was not accountable for these prior problems, but, in her efforts to manage these problems, Ms M sought to establish stricter quality control procedures and to implement the Pediatric Program within the federal guidelines and recommendations.

Social factors also affected the decision-making process. Ms M's decision was colored by her lack of experience in her position and Dr X's entrenchment and connections to his superiors in the State Health Department. She was also concerned about Dr X's numerous personal comments about her longevity in the job. Due to this, Ms M sought to reinstate compliance with federal regulations rather than reporting or directly censuring Dr X's unprofessional behavior. She did create a safety net whereby Dr X, should he continue not to follow administrative procedures, would receive reprimands and potentially lose his job.

Quality of Decision and Course of Action

Ms M's decision was to institute two new policies for the distribution of funding from the Division of Primary Care: (1) Distribution of funds was to be contingent on the submission of monthly data by each agency; and (2) all agencies were to be evaluated at monthly intervals. The purpose of these contingencies was to make certain that monies were justly spent, or more specifically, that the indigent children received what they deserved. Ms M adopted a utilitarian approach in that she sought to maximize benefits and minimize harm for the children, herself, and Dr X. Ms M made a conscious choice not to inform the authorities about Dr X's questionable spending in order to allow the indigent children to continue to receive the funds they were due.

This course of action was morally justified according to the principle of justice because each child obtained what was due him or her. This principle was based on the morally relevant properties of right and need. The children had a right to the pediatric services and had a clear need for these services. This course of action was also justified according to the principle of beneficence in that the actions taken benefitted the children who needed the care. As the elderly did not benefit from this decision, Ms M began to collect data and to work with Dr X to communicate their needs to the Director of the Health Department.

REFLECTION ON DECISION
AND COURSE OF ACTION

V. Reflection on Decision and Course of Action
   A. Reflection on Decision
      1. Was the decision that was made the one that was actually acted upon? If not, why not?
      2. Did the decision that was made accomplish its intended purpose? If not, why not?
      3. In retrospect, do you believe the decision that was made was morally good or right? Why? Why not?
   B. Reflection on Course of Action
      1. Was the selected course of action carried out in the manner intended? If not, why not?
      2. Did the selected course of action accomplish its intended purpose? If not, why not?
      3. In retrospect, do you believe the course of action taken was morally good or right? Why? Why not?

Ms M acted upon her decision to implement new policies and procedures regarding the distribution of monies in the Division of Primary Care. Through these administrative measures, she achieved her goal of delivering health care services to the persons in need in District

X and more generally throughout the state. This decision was morally right because it enabled the children in District X to obtain the services they needed and deserved, it enabled Ms M to monitor the delivery of care and spending patterns of Agency X, it gave Dr X an opportunity to correct his unprofessional behavior, and it opened the door for possible funding for the elderly in District X.

The selected course of action was carried out, and this action did accomplish Ms M's goal of providing care to those in need. The course of action taken, from a utilitarian perspective, led to the greatest good (health care for children) for the greatest number (the children, Ms M, Dr X). As the utilitarian approach in this case created some injustice for the elderly minority, Ms M sought to represent the needs of this group to Health Department authorities.

From a deontological perspective, the moral duty to deliver the health care to the children outweighed the duty to confront and report Dr X's activities. Ms M's solution struck at the core of the problem, maintaining the integrity of pediatric services for the indigent children and working to improve the administrative management of Agency X, so that the needs of the elderly could also be met within appropriate policies.

CASE COMMENTARY[6]

As a new administrator in the Division of Primary Care, it was difficult to sort out the best approach to take for the children who needed and deserved the pediatric service. I was concerned about the improper administrative procedures being used by Dr X and his staff as these procedures could potentially be questioned from a legal perspective. Since I was accountable for this Division, I also sought to stop improper actions by Dr X and his staff. My goals were to assure that the children received the care they were due and to develop an evaluation system that would enable me to confront Dr X and his staff using due process.

Staff errors and limitations frequently create ethical dilemmas in the workplace. How the administrator confronts these ethical challenges is dependent on her ethical principles and moral justification of these principles. I did not believe that explaining the errors to Dr X would have produced the desired results. This approach was too simplistic and did not take into account social

[6]Case Commentary by: **Janet L. Chapin, RN, MPH,** Administrator, Underserved Women, American College of Obstetricians and Gynecologists, Washington, D.C.

and political factors. It seemed to me that what was needed was an account-ability system that included, but was not limited to, Dr X.

It was interesting to rethink this complex case within the parameters of a systematic framework. Generally, there is no time for this type of analysis in the middle of a controversy. Nevertheless, at the time, my approach to the case was determined by two goals: (1) getting the children the services they were due and (2) maintaining personal and professional integrity for myself and those I supervised.

Although the ethical analysis was paramount in this case, I felt it was possible to be morally right and still be unable to implement the desired outcome (pediatric services for the indigent children) alone. Since there wasn't enough power within the Division, nor did I have the personal power to accomplish the change alone, I harnessed the support of a significant group of allies throughout the Health Department. The strategy was developed to in-clude others, particularly peers of Dr X, to induce Dr X and his staff to change their practices.

The strategy I selected was moderately successful. There were changes and improvements in the administrative activities at Agency X but not as many as I had hoped. Most importantly, Dr X and his staff did comply with federal regulations, spending the funds solely on the Pediatric Program. Although Dr X sought to enlist support for development of the home care program for the elderly, no state or federal program funds were allocated. It was my assessment that Dr X continued to need monitoring and supervision in the area of admin-istrative policy and procedures to prevent any other occurrences of similar activities. Through this situation, I learned that the combination of careful, reasoned analysis of the ethical issues, combined with negotiation and problem-solving skills, could be successful at producing the most desired outcome.

This case has illustrated the principle of justice as fairness and/or equality, which is a fundamental concept in program administration. As was evident in this case, there are no easy answers to ethical dilemmas concerning justice. Rather, it is important that nurse administrators consider factors contributing to the dilemmas and then determine approaches to resolving these dilemmas that can be morally justified.

___

Summary. This case represents a retrospective analysis of the interplay among the ethical principles of justice and beneficence. The principle of justice provides the basis for the moral justification for an ethical dilemma about the distribution of funds and health care to individuals who deserved the services (the children) and those who needed the services (the children and the elderly). Using a utilitarian and a deontological perspective, the decision-making process and course of action were examined, and the moral justification for the decision was presented. Finally, the nurse/health care administrator who dealt with the case comments upon the analysis in retrospect.

REFERENCES

Beauchamp, T. L. (1982). *Philosophical ethics: An introduction to moral philosophy.* New York: McGraw–Hill.

Mill, J. S. (1979). *Utilitarianism* (G. Sher, Ed.). Indianapolis: Hackett. (Original work published 1861)

Epilogue

The purpose of this book is to increase nurse administrators' knowledge about and self-confidence in resolving ethical dilemmas. To that end, the book combines both theory and application. The theory provides nurse administrators with basic knowledge about ethical theories, principles, and moral development. The application provides nurse administrators with a framework for systematic analyses of administrative ethical dilemmas.

The preceding understanding of basic moral philosophy and systematic analyses is important because it provides nurse administrators with a relatively stable knowledge base and framework for examining ethical issues. Such a knowledge base and framework are important, particularly in times like these when new ethical dilemmas arise daily. With few modifications, the knowledge base and framework described in this book should help nurse administrators to examine ethical dilemmas they face now and in the immediate future.

The Ethics of Nursing: A Selected Bibliography

Doris Mueller Goldstein

The primary purpose of this bibliography is to provide the reader with an overview of contemporary literature on nursing ethics. Priority has been given to recent substantive works authored by nurses, but there are exceptions to this. All of the citations are to English-language works, and some of the books are accompanied by brief annotations.

Information in various formats has been included, ranging from audiovisual materials to dissertations. Although many of these materials are part of collections of the National Reference Center for Bioethics Literature, some documents must be obtained from other sources. Since the National Reference Center will continue to collect writings such as these in the future, your comments regarding items omitted or erroneously cited would be appreciated by the compiler, who takes full responsibility for any inaccuracies in this document.

The major portion of this bibliography is devoted to book and journal literature. Five subject-oriented subdivisions have been used to categorize these writings: general and philosophical writings, codes of nursing ethics, ethics and nursing education, ethics and nursing practice, and ethics and nursing research. Within each group, arrangement is alphabetical by author.

Tools helpful for working with this literature, as well as tools for maintaining currency in the field, are also suggested.

One unique feature of this bibliography is the section on dissertations in nursing ethics. A computer search was made of the Dissertation Abstracts International database for research on nursing ethics, and 90 dissertations were selected for inclusion here. Order is alphabetical by author. Copies of most of these dissertations can be obtained from University Microfilms International, Ann Arbor, Michigan; the required order number is included with each citation. It is hoped that this listing might aid the germination of ideas for further research as well as lessen redundant efforts.

In addition to the dissertations, two segments are devoted to specialized forms of information that merit separate listing: bibliographies and audiovisual materials.

AN INTRODUCTION TO ETHICS

Four of the five works below can serve as a basic introductory text for becoming familiar with ethical theories, and the fifth, by Goldman, provides an analysis of the underpinnings of professional ethics.

Beauchamp, Tom L. *Philosophical Ethics: An Introduction to Moral Philosophy.* New York: McGraw–Hill, 1982. 396 pp.

Frankena, William K. *Ethics* (2nd ed.). Englewood Cliffs, NJ: Prentice-Hall, 1973. 144 pp.

Goldman, Alan H. *The Moral Foundations of Professional Ethics.* Totowa, NJ: Rowman and Littlefield, 1980. 305 pp.

Rachels, James. *The Elements of Moral Philosophy.* Philadelphia: Temple University Press, 1986. 169 pp.

Taylor, Paul W. *Principles of Ethics: An Introduction.* Encino, CA: Dickenson Publishing Co., 1975. 234 pp.

AN INTRODUCTION TO BIOETHICS

The following books provide broad overviews of the field of bioethics. One comprehensive reference work, by Reich, is also cited.

Beauchamp, Tom L., & Childress, James. *Principles of Biomedical Ethics* (3rd ed.). New York: Oxford University Press, 1989. 454 pp.

Beauchamp, Tom L., & Walters, LeRoy (Comps.). *Contemporary Issues in Bioethics* (3rd ed.). Belmont, CA: Wadsworth Publishing Co., 1989. 655 pp.

Jonsen, Albert R.; Siegler, Mark; & Winslade, William J. *Clinical Ethics: A Practical Approach to Ethical Decisions in Clinical Medicine* (2nd ed.). New York: Macmillan, 1986. 202 pp.

Levine, Carol. *Taking Sides: Clashing Views on Controversial Bioethical Issues* (3rd ed.). Guilford, CT: Dushkin Publishing Group, 1989. 96 pp.

Levine, Carol, & Veatch, Robert M. (Eds.). *Cases in Bioethics from the Hastings Center Report.* Hastings–on–Hudson, NY: Hastings Center, 1984. 127 pp.

Mappes, Thomas A., & Zembaty, Jane S. (Eds.). *Biomedical Ethics* (2nd ed.). New York: McGraw–Hill, 1986. 657 pp.

Reich, Warren T. (Ed.). *Encyclopedia of Bioethics.* New York: Free Press, 1978. Four volumes; 1933 pp. (Reissued in two volumes in 1982)

Veatch, Robert M. *Medical Ethics.* Boston: Jones and Bartlett, 1989. 372 pp.

Hospital ethics committees have emerged as an increasingly common institutional entity throughout the United States. Since nurses are frequently asked to serve as committee members, four citations have been included here to provide information in support of this new role.

Cranford, R. E., & Doudera, A. E. *Institutional Ethics Committees and Health Care Decision Making.* Ann Arbor, MI: Health Administration Press, 1984. 424 pp.

Hosford, Bowen. *Bioethics Committees: The Health Care Provider's Guide.* Rockville, MD: Aspen Systems Corp., 1986. 340 pp.

McCarrick, Pat Milmoe. *Ethics Committees in Hospitals.* Washington, DC: Kennedy Institute of Ethics, Georgetown University, June 1989. 12 pp. (Scope Note No. 3, revised)

Ross, J. W. *Handbook for Hospital Ethics Committees.* Chicago: American Hospital Publishing Co., 1986. 164 pp.

FORMAT-ORIENTED CITATIONS IN NURSING ETHICS

Dissertations in Nursing Ethics from 1970 to the Present

Due to the magnitude of research in bioethical issues at the graduate level, this list is limited to dissertations that deal primarily with nursing ethics.

Allen, Carol Maureen Easley. "Holism and Nursing: An Analysis of the Pragmatic Consequences of a Theoretical Concept for a Helping Profession." New York University, Ph.D. diss., 1983. 307 pp. University Microfilms Order No. ADG84–12326.

Applegate, Minerva Irons. "Moral Decisions in Selected Clinical Nursing Practice Situations." Columbia University Teachers College, Ed.D. diss., 1981. 154 pp. University Microfilms Order No. ADG81–22930.

Aronovitz, Frances Britton. "Autonomy, Socialization, Strength of Religious Belief and Socioeconomic Status as Predictors of Moral Judgement in Associate Degree Nursing Students University of Miami." University of Miami, Ph.D. diss., 1984. 148 pp. University Microfilms Order No. ADG85–06550.

Awtrey, Janet Shealy. "Moral Reasoning of Baccalaureate Nursing Students." University of Alabama in Birmingham, D.S.N. diss., 1980. 102 pp. University Microfilms Order No. ADG81–12733.

Babcock, Patricia Ann. "The Nurse and Euthanasia." Ball State University, Ed.D. diss., 1980. 132 pp. University Microfilms Order No. ADG81–04880.

Beardslee, Nancy Quinn. "Survey of Teaching Ethics in Nursing Programs and the Investigation of the Relationship Between Extent of Ethics Content and Moral Reasoning Levels." University of Northern Colorado, Ed.D. diss., 1983. 111 pp. University Microfilms Order No. ADG83–24326.

Beauregard, Florence Elaine. "Educational Level and Moral Development of Intensive Care Nurses." Texas Woman's University, M.S. thesis, 1983. 68 pp. University Microfilms Order No. ADG13–21325.

Bell, Carolyn M. Webb. "Adult Life Crises, Sexism, and Moral Reasoning in Female Nurses." Texas Woman's University, Ph.D. diss., 1983. 156 pp. University Microfilms Order No. ADG84–09204.

Bell, Shirley Kay. "Effect of a Biomedical Ethics Course on Senior Nursing Students' Level of Moral Development." West Virginia University, Ed.D. diss., 1984. 108 pp. University Microfilms Order No. ADG84–29854.

Benner, Margaret Patricia. "Value Pluralism, Moral Competence, and Nursing Education." University of Delaware, Ph.D. diss., 1985. 217 pp. University Microfilms Order No. AAD85–11222.

Berry, Margaret Ann Jennings. "Opinions of Oklahoma Registered Nurses Regarding Health Services for Minors Without Parental Consent or Knowledge." Oklahoma State University, Ph.D. diss., 1982. 171 pp. University Microfilms Order No. ADG83–00137.

Biehler, Barbara Ann. "Using Instructional Design to Resolve a Problem in Teaching Ethics to Baccalaureate Nursing Students." Illinois State University, Ed.D. diss., 1986. 230 pp. University Microfilms Order No. AAD87–05737.

Breslin, Eileen. "Health Beliefs of Female Artists Concerning Reproductive Occupational Health Hazards." University of Arizona, M.S. thesis, 1983. 112 pp. University Microfilms Order No. ADG13–21426.

Capp, Sheila Putman. "The Effects of Selected Hospital Milieu Factors on the Levels of Moral Reasoning in Nurses." University of Missouri–Columbia, M.S. thesis, 1984. 94 pp. University Microfilms Order No. ADG13–24263.

Chambliss, Daniel Frederick. "The Bounds of Responsibility: A Study in the Social Psychology of Nursing Ethics." Yale University, Ph.D. diss., 1982. 172 pp. University Microfilms Order No. AAD82–20829.

Cochran, Ruth Beardsley. "Some Problems with Loyalty: With Special Application to Nursing Ethics." University of Colorado at Boulder, Ph.D. diss., 1985. 148 pp. University Microfilms Order No. ADG86–08593.

Copstead, Lee-Ellen Charlotte. "An Examination of Relationships: Perceived Normative Ethical Stance/Perceived Realistic Ethical Choice and Self-Esteem Among Selected Groups of Registered Nurses in Washington State." Gonzaga University, Ed.D. diss., 1983. 134 pp. University Microfilms Order No. AAD84–03908.

Cox, Jonathon Lawrence. "Ethical Decision Making by Hospital Nurses." Wayne State University, Ph.D. diss., 1985. 96 pp. University Microfilms Order No. ADG86–04989.

Crisham, Patricia. "Moral Judgment of Nurses in Hypothetical and Nursing Dilemmas." University of Minnesota, Ph.D. diss., 1979. 144 pp. University Microfilms Order No. ADG80–06598.

De Jong, Ann Frances. "The Relationship of Moral Reasoning and Perceived Autonomy at Work to Ethical Judgment Among Female Registered Nurses." New York University, Ph.D. diss., 1984. 99 pp. University Microfilms Order No. ADG85–05415.

Dison, Norma Jean. "Dilemmas of Baccalaureate Nursing Students." University of Minnesota, Ph.D. diss., 1985. 262 pp. University Microfilms Order No. ADG85–26469.

Durkis, Joan Michele. "The Development of Administrative Considerations for the Placement of Staff Nurses in Reference to Death and the Dying Patient." Florida Atlantic University, Ed.D. diss., 1982. 547 pp. University Microfilms Order No. ADG82–15565.

Eberhardy, Jeanette Luise. "An Analysis of Moral Decision Making with Nursing Students Facing Professional Problems." University of Minnesota, Ph.D. diss., 1982. 128 pp. University Microfilms Order No. AAD83–08040.

Edgil, Ann Estes. "Variables Related to the Principled Level of Moral Judgment of Nurses." University of Alabama in Birmingham, D.S.N. diss., 1980. 102 pp. University Microfilms Order No. ADG81–12734.

Eschbach, Delphine Muriel Wentland. "An Investigation of the Reasons Why Nurses Accept and Continue Employment in Positions in Lingering Dying Trajectory Settings." University of California, San Francisco, D.N.S. diss., 1980. 163 pp. University Microfilms Order No. ADG81–04448.

Felton, Gwen McCarter. "Attribution of Responsibility, Ethical/Moral Reasoning and the Ability of Undergraduate and Graduate Nursing Students to Resolve Ethical/Moral Dilemmas." University of South Carolina, Ph.D. diss., 1984. 163 pp. University Microfilms Order No. ADG85–08176.

Finch, A. Joyce. "Relationship Between Organizational Climate and Nurses' Ethical Decisions." University of Texas at Austin, Ph.D. diss., 1986. 290 pp. University Microfilms Order No. ADG86–18466.

Firlit, Sharon Louise. "Consensus and Outcome of a Philosophy of Nursing Belief: Patient as the Primary Decision Maker." University of Illinois at Chicago, Health Sciences Center, Ph.D. diss., 1983. 224 pp. University Microfilms Order No. ADG83–20381.

Fleeger, Rebekah L. "Critical Thinking and Moral Reasoning Behavior of Baccalaureate Nursing Students." Claremont Graduate School, Ph.D. diss., 1986. 208 pp. University Microfilms Order No. AAD86–16530.

Fowler, Marsha Diane Mary. "Ethics and Nursing, 1893-1984: The Ideal of Service, The Reality of History." University of Southern California, Ph.D. diss., 1984. 420 l. (Not available from University Microfilms International.)

Frisch, Noreen Cavan. "The Value Analysis Model and the Moral and Cognitive Development of Baccalaureate Nursing Students." Southern Illinois University at Carbondale, Ph.D. diss., 1986. 127 pp. University Microfilms Order No. ADG86–22978.

Fry, Sara Thomson. "Protecting Privacy: Judicial Decision-Making in Search of a Principle." Georgetown University, Ph.D. diss., 1984. 179 pp. University Microfilms Order No. AAD85–27453.

Gale, Elizabeth Jeannine Masden. "Perceptions of Counselees Seeking Mid-Trimester Prenatal Diagnosis." Indiana University School of Nursing D.N.S. diss., 1983. 220 pp. University Microfilms Order No. ADG84, 00848.

Garritson, Susan Hunn. "The Influence of Psychiatric Inpatient Environments on Ethical Decision Making of Psychiatric Nurses." University of California, San Francisco, D.N.S. diss., 1985. 187 pp. University Microfilms Order No. ADG85-24004.

Gaul, Alice Leveille. "Moral Reasoning and Ethical Decision Making in Nursing Practice." Texas Woman's University, Ph.D. diss., 1986. 155 pp. University Microfilms Order No. ADG86-26482.

Giovinco, Gina. "Using Patient Care Situations to Apply Kohlberg's Moral Development Theory to Nursing." Temple University, Ed.D. diss., 1985. 121 pp. University Microfilms Order No. AAD85-21084.

Holly, Cheryl Malahan. "Staff Nurses' Participation in Ethical Decision Making: A Descriptive Study of Selected Situational Variables." Columbia University Teachers College, Ed.D. diss., 1986. 182 pp. University Microfilms Order No. ADG86-20367.

Holzman, Phyllis Gollin. "A Comparative Study of Liberal Arts and Nursing Students' Moral Development in Collegiate Programs." Marquette University, Ph.D. diss., 1984. 97 pp. University Microfilms Order No. ADG85-02589.

Horan, Mary L. Fussman. "The Relationship Between Parental Attributions and Adjustment to the Birth of an Infant with a Defect." University of Michigan, Ph.D. diss., 1983. 145 pp. University Microfilms Order No. ADG84-02295.

Howe, Kenneth Ross. "Evaluating Medical Ethics Teaching." Michigan State University, Ph.D. diss., 1985. 251 pp. University Microfilms Order No. AAD85-20529.

Johnson, Rosalind Winifred Heyward. "A Comparison of the Perceptions among Student Nurses from Associate Degree, Baccalaureate and Diploma Programs in Nursing about the Influence of Significant Others and the Curriculum upon the Moral/Ethical Component of the Professional Role." State University of New York at Albany, Ed.D. diss., 1980. 225 pp. University Microfilms Order No. ADG80-18423.

Jones, Maxine Blackmon. "A Case Analysis of the Legal, Professional, and Ethical Responsibilities of Registered Nurses for Disclosure of Prognostic Information to Dying Adults." University of Alabama in Birmingham, D.S.N. diss., 1983. 199 pp. University Microfilms Order No. ADG84-14554.

Keller, Marjorie C. "Nurses' Responses to Moral Dilemmas." University of South Carolina, Ed.D. diss., 1985. 147 pp. University Microfilms Order No. ADG85-18030.

Kellmer, Dorothy Margaret. "The Teaching of Ethical Decision Making in Schools of Nursing: Variables and Strategies." Gonzaga University, Ed.D. diss., 1984. 218 pp. University Microfilms Order No. ADG84-16265.

Kowalski, Jo Anne Theresa. "An Investigation into the Phenomenon of Caring Within the Nursing Experience." Boston University, Ed.D. diss., 1985. 269 pp. University Microfilms Order No. ADG86–01353.

Krawczyk, Rosemary Margaret. "Moral Judgment Level of Nursing Students in Three Different Nursing Programs." Boston College, Ph.D. diss., 1982. 126 pp. University Microfilms Order No. AAD82–15657.

Krizinofski, Marian Theresa Lesko. "A Conceptual Foundation for Nursing Ethics." Syracuse University, Ph.D. diss., 1984. 263 pp. University Microfilms Order No. ADG85–01715.

Kudzma, Elizabeth Anne Connelly. "Moral Reasoning of Nurses in the Work Setting." Boston University School of Nursing, D.N.Sc. diss., 1980. 166 pp. University Microfilms Order No. ADG80–24233.

Kurman, Elaine Cooper. "Nurses' Attitudes Toward Passive Euthanasia for the Severely Handicapped Child." Columbia University Teachers College, Ed.D. diss., 1984. 255 pp. University Microfilms Order No. ADG84–11274.

Lamb, M. "Nursing Ethics in Canada: Two Decades." University of Alberta, Master's thesis, 1981. (Not available from University Microfilms International.)

Lazerine, Neil G. "Professional Perspectives on Euthanasia: A Comparative Study of Nurses and Clergymen." Bowling Green State University, Ph.D. diss., 1977. 387 pp. University Microfilms Order No. 78–232.

Lentz, Mary Elizabeth. "Congruency of Nurses' Perceptions of Responsibility and Accountability with Professional Expectations for Clinical Practice." University of Pittsburgh, Ph.D. diss., 1985. 124 pp. University Microfilms Order No. ADG86–02806.

Levy, Suzanne Bryer. "An Analysis of Helping Models and Helping Behaviors in a Group of Psychiatric Nurses." University of Pennsylvania, Ph.D. diss., 1986. 114 pp. University Microfilms Order No. ADG86–14827.

Mahon, Kathleen Ann. "Constructs Used by Registered Nurses in Ethical Decision Making: The Development of an Instrument." University of San Francisco, Ed.D. diss., 1981. 148 pp. University Microfilms Order No. AAD81–20481.

Matthews, Anne Lamphier. "A Developmental Process of Loss: The Impact of Known Fetal Malformations on Pregnant Women Evaluated by a Fetal Medicine and Surgery Program." University of Colorado Health Sciences Center, Ph.D. diss., 1984. 317 pp. University Microfilms Order No. ADG84–28940.

Mayberry, M. Adrienne. "Moral Reasoning in Ethical Dilemmas of Staff Nurses and Head Nurses." University of Southern California, D.P.A. diss., 1983. (Not available from University Microfilms International.)

Mooney, Mary Margaret. "The Code for Nurses: A Survey of Its Content, Constitutive Structure, and Usefulness to the Nursing Profession." The Catholic University of America, D.N.Sc. diss., 1980. 176 pp. University Microfilms Order No. ADG80–18912.

Munhall, Patricia Lynn. "Moral Reasoning Levels of Nursing Students and Faculty in a Baccalaureate Nursing Program." Columbia University Teachers College, Ed.D. diss., 1979. 227 pp. University Microfilms Order No. ADG80–06842.

Murphy, Catherine Patricia. "Levels of Moral Reasoning in a Selected Group of Nursing Practitioners." Columbia University Teachers College, Ed.D. diss., 1976. 178 pp. University Microfilms Order No. ADG77–16684.

Mustapha, Sherry Lee Wells. "An Examination of Moral Reasoning in College Students in Two Types of General Education Curricula: Implications for Nursing Education." University of Kansas, Ed.D. diss., 1985. 130 pp. University Microfilms Order No. ADG86–08467.

Noffsinger, Anne Russell Lillis. "American and British Nurses' Attitudes Toward Disabled Persons: The Role of Needs and Moral Reasoning." University of Kentucky, Ed.D. diss., 1979. 150 pp. University Microfilms Order No. ADG79–27706.

Nokes, Kathleen Mary. "The Relationship Between Moral Reasoning, the Relationship Dimension of the Social Climate of the Work Environment, and Perception of Realistic Moral Behavior Among Registered Professional Nurses." New York University, Ph.D. diss., 1985. 114 pp. University Microfilms Order No. ADG85–10768.

Obester, Dorothy Mae. "The Place of Ethics as an Area of Study in the Curricula of Schools of Nursing in Pennsylvania." University of Pittsburgh, Ph.D. diss., 1985. 117 pp. University Microfilms Order No. ADG86–17243.

Omery, Anna Kathryn. "The Moral Reasoning of Nurses Who Work in the Adult Intensive Care Setting." Boston University, D.N.Sc. diss., 1985. 182 pp. University Microfilms Order No. ADG85–24191.

Paterson, Josephine G. "Echo Into Tomorrow: A Mental Health Psychiatric Philosophical Conceptualization of Nursing." Boston University School of Nursing, D.N.Sc. diss., 1969. 115 pp. University Microfilms Order No. ADG70–01039.

Payton, Rita Jean. "A Bioethical Program of Study for Baccalaureate Nursing Students." University of Northern Colorado, D.A. diss., 1978. 122 pp. University Microfilms Order No. 79–10311.

Penny, Jean Tredinick. "A Comparison of Faculty and Nurse Practitioner Opinions Regarding Practice Issues, Political Education, and Professional Ethics." Florida State University, Ph.D. diss., 1983. 188 pp. University Microfilms Order No. AAD83–14196.

Peterson, Marjory. "The Norms and Values Held by Three Groups of Nurses Concerning Psychosocial Nursing Practice." Columbia University Teachers College, Ed.D. diss., 1985. 203 pp. University Microfilms Order No. ADG86–02.

Pierce, Cheryl Denise. "An Assessment of Ethical Dilemmas Known to Mental Health Professionals." University of Pittsburgh, Ph.D. diss., 1985. 275 pp. University Microfilms Order No. AAD86–02811.

Pinch, Winifred Jane. "Ethical and Moral Dilemmas in Nursing: The Role of the Nurse and Perceptions of Autonomy." Boston University School of Education, Ed.D. diss., 1983. 303 pp. University Microfilms Order No. ADG83–19931.

Polk, Glenda Chitwood. "A Comparison of Crisis Variables Among Groups of Women Experiencing Induced Abortion." University of Alabama in Birmingham, D.S.N. diss., 1983. 314 pp. University Microfilms Order No. ADG84–04471.

Praeger, Susan Gray. "Humanistic Nursing Education: Considerations and Proposals." University of Northern Colorado, Ed.D. diss., 1980. 145 pp. University Microfilms Order No. ADG80–28346.

Preheim, Gayle Gullickson. "Perspectives in Psycho-Ethical Decision Making: Implications for Collaboration Between Nursing Education and Practice." University of South Dakota, Ed.D. diss., 1985. 278 pp. University Microfilms Order No. ADG85–14220.

Rasor, Beverly Ann Boykin. "Moral Judgment: A Comparison Between Hospital and Public Health Nurses." Texas Woman's University, M.S. thesis, 1982. 73 pp. University Microfilms Order No. ADG13–20570.

Reisman, Elizabeth Cornman. "Recall of the Process of Informed Consent as Perceived by Patient–Subjects, Physician Researchers, and Professional Nurses." The Catholic University of America, D.N.Sc. diss., 1985. 327 pp. University Microfilms Order No. AAD85–15049.

Risser, Joy. "The Hospice Kind of Care: A Work of Love." University of California, Los Angeles, Ph.D. diss., 1984. 141 pp. University Microfilms Order No. AAD85–05665.

Rorer, Brett Allan. "Interactions Between Patients and Nurses During Hemodialysis." University of Florida, Ph.D. diss., 1986. 116 pp. University Microfilms Order No. ADG86–18671.

Saarmann, Lembi. "Ideals for Nurses: A Study of the 'American Journal of Nursing' and 'RN', 1940–1960." Columbia University Teachers College, Ed.D. diss., 1986. 269 pp. University Microfilms Order No. ADG86–11698.

Sleicher, Martha Neff. "Moral Judgments: A Study Investigating Instrument Development for The Nursing Profession." University of Michigan, Ph.D. diss., 1978. 135 pp. University Microfilms Order No. ADG78–23010.

Smith, Aaron Anthony. "Mothers of Life-Agent Strategists in Neonatal Intensive Care Nurseries." University of California, San Francisco, Ph.D. diss., 1984. 307 pp. University Microfilms Order No. AAD85–13665.

Smith, Elizabeth Dorsey Ivey. "Attitudes Among Baccalaureate Nursing Students in New York City Regarding Women Seeking Elective Abortions." Columbia University Teachers College, Ed.D. diss., 1975. 125 pp. University Microfilms Order No. ADG76–03274.

Smith, Mary Columbus. "Baccalaureate Nursing Students' Attitudes Toward Abortion." Texas Southern University, Ed.D. diss., 1985. 98 pp. University Microfilms Order No. AAD85–29601.

Smith, Sharon Jeanne. "Directions for a New Discipline: Knowing, Meaning and Value in the Conceptualization of a Body of Knowledge for Nursing." Graduate Theological Union, Ph.D. diss., 1983. 234 pp. University Microfilms Order No. ADG83–28369.

Swanson, Kauffman Kristen M. "The Unborn One: A Profile of the Human Experience of Miscarriage." University of Colorado Health Sciences Center, Ph.D. diss., 1983. 317 pp. University Microfilms Order No. ADG84–04456.

Thompson, Jacqueline K. "Women's Attitudes Towards Selected Health Issues: Implications for Nursing Education." State University of New York at Buffalo, Ph.D. diss., 1986. 374 pp. University Microfilms Order No. ADG86–29119.

Turner, Virginia Ann. "The Relationship Between Moral Judgment and Moral Action Among Professional Nurses." Fordham University, Ph.D., diss., 1984. 146 pp. University Microfilms Order No. AAD84–23138.

Walters, Marlene Louise. "An Experimental Study of the Impact of a Program on the Medical Options of Sanctity or Quality of Life upon Nursing Students." Eastern Baptist Theological Seminary, D.Min. diss., 1980. 339 pp. University Microfilms Order No. AAD80–20454.

Watanabe, Katharine Keiko. "Health Care in Transition: A Moral Order in Passage Through Social and Technological Change." University of California, San Francisco, D.N.S. diss., 1972. 269 pp. University Microfilms Order No. ADG73–06529.

Winland-Brown, Jill E. "A Comparison of Student Nurses, Nurses and Non-Nurses with Regard to Their Moral Judgments on Nursing Dilemmas." Florida Atlantic University, Ed.D. diss., 1983. 105 pp. University Microfilms Order No. ADG84–03838.

Zablow, Robin Jean. "Preparing Students for the Moral Dimension of Professional Nursing Practice: A Protocol for Nurse Educators." Columbia University Teachers College, Ed.D. diss., 1984. 178 pp. University Microfilms Order No. ADG84–24277.

Bibliographical Resources on Nursing Ethics

American Nurses' Association. *Committee on Ethics. Ethics in Nursing: References and Resources* [Kathleen M. Sward, chairperson]. Kansas City, MO: The Association, 1979. 31 pp. (See *Ethics References for Nurses below.*)

American Nurses' Association. Committee on Ethics. Ethics References for Nurses. Kansas City, MO: American Nurses' Association, 1982. 40 pp. An update of *Ethics in Nursing: References and Resources,* this unannotated bibliography is organized by nine issue-oriented subject categories. Also included are audiovisual materials and U.S. government publications.

Pence, Terry. *Ethics in Nursing: An Annotated Bibliography* (2nd ed.). New York: National League for Nursing, 1986. 255 pp.

Walters, LeRoy, & Kahn, Tamar Joy (Eds.). *Bibliography of Bioethics,* Vol 1– , 1975– (Vols. 1–6 published by Gale Research Co.; Vols. 7–9 published by Free Press, New York; and Vols. 10– published by the Kennedy Institute of Ethics, Georgetown University, Washington, DC.) This annual bibliography corresponds to the latest one-year increment to the BIO-ETHICSLINE database. Typically 2400 citations to various document types are included; these cover all aspects of bioethics. "Nursing Ethics" is a primary, regular subject heading in the *Bibliography*.

Audiovisual Resources

Most of the materials listed below, all of which are of particular interest to the nursing profession, were selected from the AVLINE online database available from the National Library of Medicine. (The Library loans these via Interlibrary Loan.) For a more complete listing of bioethics audiovisuals in general the reader may wish to consult: (1) the BIOETHICSLINE database of the National Library of Medicine or (2) *Human Values in Medicine and Health Care: Audio–Visual Resources*, compiled by Nadya Shmavonian, New Haven: Yale University Press, 1983.

Finally, the National Reference Center for Bioethics Literature published a Scope Note in 1988 entitled "Bioethics Audiovisuals, 1982 to Present," which provides a selected, annotated guide to audiovisuals in bioethics.

"Accountability and the Phases of Management." [Videorecording]. Chicago: S–N Publications, 1979. One videocassette (24 min.); sound; color; ¾ in.; includes one instructor's guide.

"Bioethics in Nursing Practice." [Videorecording]. Written by Lauraine A. Thomas. Bowie, MD: Robert J. Brady Co., 1981. Five videocassettes (76 min.); sound; color; ¾ in.; includes one guide.

"Code Gray: Ethical Dilemmas in Nursing." [Motion picture or Videorecording]. Jamaica Plain, MA: Fanlight Products, 1984. One 16 mm. film or videocassette; 28 min.; sound; color.

"Ethical–Legal Aspects of Nursing Practice." Developed by Susan R. Gortner and Doris Bloch. [Videorecording]. New York: Educational Services Division, American Journal of Nursing Company, 1974. One cassette; 30 min.; sound; color; ¾ in. [Discusses death with dignity and treatment refusal.]

"Ethics in Nursing." Presented by Mary Cipriano Silva and Tom L. Beauchamp. [Videorecording]. Fairfax, VA: School of Nursing, George Mason University, 1986. Nine videocassettes (4 hr.); sound; color; includes study guide. [Contains five units; based on a three-day ethics conference held at George Mason University and Georgetown University.]

"Ethics, Values and Health Care." [Filmstrip]. Irvine, CA: Concept Media, 1980. Eight rolls; color; 35 mm. and 8 cassettes (two-track, monaural, approximately 20 min. each); includes guide. [Covers several bioethical issues facing the nursing profession.]

"The Nurse's Responsibility and Conflicts Encountered in the Care of the Terminally Ill Patients." [Videorecording]. Marshfield, WI: The Marshfield Regional Video Network, in cooperation with Marshfield Clinic and St. Joseph's Hospital, 1981. One videocassette; 62 min.; sound; color; ¾ in.

"Parents and Children." [Videorecording]. New York: American Journal of
Nursing Co., Education Services Division; for loan by Modern Talking
Picture Services, Inc., St. Petersburg, FL; 1977. One cassette, 30 min.;
sound; color; ¾ inch; includes guide. [Covers informed consent and
minors.]
"Professional Ethics." [Filmstrip]. Tulsa, OK: Health Media Corp., in cooperation with Hillcrest Medical Center, Tulsa, OK; for loan and sale by Trainex
Corp., Garden Grove, CA; 1978. 102 frames; color; 35 mm. and cassette
(two-track, monaural, 17 min.); includes guide.

SUBJECT-ORIENTED CITATIONS
IN NURSING ETHICS (BOOKS AND ARTICLES)

General and Philosophical Writings

"A *Nursing Life* Poll Report on Ethics: How Ethical Are You? Part 2." *Nursing
Life* 3 (1983): 46–56.
American Nurses' Association. Committee on Ethics. Ethical Dilemmas Confronting Nurses. Kansas City, MO: American Nurses' Association (2420
Pershing Rd., Kansas City, MO 64108), 1985. 30 pp. Reprints of brief
articles previously published between November 1983 and September
1984 in *The American Nurse*, these essays address such topics as foregoing
treatment and the allocation of scarce resources.
American Nurses' Association. Committee on Ethics. *Ethics in Nursing Practice
and Education.* Kansas City, MO: American Nurses' Association, 1980. 65
pp. Originally presented at the ANA Convention held in Houston June 8–
13, 1980, these seven papers address ethics in nursing practice and in
nursing education.
Aroskar, Mila A. "Anatomy of an Ethical Dilemma: The Practice." *American
Journal of Nursing* 80 (1980): 661–663.
Aroskar, Mila A. "Anatomy of an Ethical Dilemma: The Theory." *American
Journal of Nursing* 80 (1980): 658–660.
Aroskar, Mila A. "Using Ethical Reasoning to Guide Clinical Decision Mak-
ing." *Perioperative Nursing Quarterly* 2 (1986): 20–26.
Bandman, Bertram. "The Role and Justification of Rights in Nursing." *Medicine
and Law* 3 (1984): 77–87.
Bandman, Elsie L., & Bandman, Bertram. *Nursing Ethics in the Life Span.*
Norwalk, CT: Appleton–Century–Crofts, 1985. 290 pp.
Benjamin, Martin, & Curtis, Joy. *Ethics in Nursing* (2nd ed.). New York: Oxford
University Press, 1986. 206 pp.
Benoliel, Jeanne Quint. "Ethics in Nursing Practice and Education." *Nursing
Outlook* 31 (1983): 210–215.
Buckenham, June E., & McGrath, Gerry. *The Social Reality of Nursing.* Boston:
Health Science Press, 1983. 110 pp.

Carmi, A., & Schneider, S. (Eds.). *Nursing Law and Ethics.* New York: Springer, 1985. 245 pp. (Medicolegal Library, No. 4)

Chinn, Peggy L. (Ed.). *Ethical Issues in Nursing.* Rockville, MD: Aspen Systems Corp., 1986. 234 pp. A collection of articles from *Advances in Nursing Science* and *Topics in Clinical Nursing.*

Chinn, Peggy L. (Ed.). *Ethics and Values.* Germantown, MD: Aspen Systems, 1979. 106 pp. (*Advances in Nursing Science 1:* 3).

Cowart, Marie E., & Allen, Rodney F. (Eds.). *Changing Conceptions of Health Care: Public Policy and Ethical Issues for Nurses.* Thorofare, NJ: C. B. Slack, 1981. 115 pp.

Crowder, Eleanor. "Manners, Morals, and Nurses: An Historical Overview of Nursing Ethics." *Texas Reports on Biology and Medicine* **32**(1): 173–180, Spring 1974.

Curtin, Leah, & Flaherty, M. Josephine. *Nursing Ethics: Theories and Pragmatics.* Bowie, MD: Brady, 1982. 363 pp.

Davis, Anne J. (Guest Ed.). "Special Issue: Ethics in Nursing." *International Journal of Nursing Studies* 22(4) (1985): 293–339. Contributors from Australia, Israel, Japan, Switzerland, and the United States examine ethical issues in nursing from different perspectives.

Davis, Anne J., & Krueger, Janelle C. (Eds.). *Patients, Nurses, Ethics.* New York: American Journal of Nursing Co., Educational Services Division, 1980. 245 pp. Includes papers presented at the 1979 Annual Meeting of the Western Society of Nurse Researchers, held in Portland, OR.

Densford, Katharine J., & Everett, Millard S. *Ethics for Modern Nurses.* New York: Garland, 1984. 260 pp. (The History of American Nursing.) Reprint of work originally published by Saunders (Philadelphia), 1946.

Ethical Issues in Nursing: A Proceedings. Adapted from nursing institutes held in Boston, Chicago, Houston, and San Francisco during 1975–1976 and sponsored by School of Nursing, Catholic University of America, Washington, DC and Department of Nursing Services, the Catholic Hospital Association, St. Louis, MO. St. Louis: Catholic Hospital Association, 1976. 99 pp.

Ethical Issues in Nursing and Nursing Education. New York: National League for Nursing, 1980. 72 pp. (Publications; National League for Nursing; No. 16–1822) Four papers from a workshop held in Washington, DC, February 21–22, 1980, are followed by guidelines for discussion.

Fenner, Kathleen M. *Ethics and Law in Nursing: Professional Perspectives.* New York: Van Nostrand Reinhold, 1980. 210 pp. Introductory chapters cover ethics, ethical codes, and the origins of personal values and the effect of these values on nursing. Then the author examines, with a case study approach, legal issues in nursing as well as specific health care issues having moral components.

Fowler, Marsha D. M. "Chirurgery: An Ethical Commentary on Surgical Technology and the Allocation of Surgical Resources." *Perioperative Nursing Quarterly* 2 (1986): 35–41, 47.

Fowler, Marsha D. M., & Levine-Ariff, June. *Ethics at the Bedside: A Source Book for the Critical Care Nurse.* Philadelphia: J. B. Lippincott, 1987. 270 pp.

Fromer, Margot Joan. *Ethical Issues in Health Care.* St. Louis: Mosby, 1981. 420 pp.

Fry, Sara T. "Ethical Principles in Nursing Education and Practice: A Missing Link in the Unification Issue." *Nursing and Health Care 3* (1982): 363–368.

Fry, Sara T. "Moral Values and Ethical Decisions in a Constrained Economic Environment." *Nursing Economic$ 4* (1986): 160–164.

Gadow, Sally. "Basis for Nursing Ethics: Paternalism, Consumerism, or Advocacy?" *Hospital Progress 64* (1983): 62–67, 78.

Georges, Jane Marie. "Ethical Issues in Perioperative Nursing Practice." *Perioperative Nursing Quarterly 2* (1986): 13–19.

Gillon, Raanan. "Nursing Ethics and Medical Ethics" [Editorial]. *Journal of Medical Ethics 12* (1986): 115–116, 122.

Gortner, Susan R. "Ethical Inquiry." In Harriet H. Werley and Fitzpatrick, Joyce J. (Eds.), *Annual Review of Nursing Research*, Vol. 3. New York: Springer, 1985; pp. 193–214. This review essay addresses specifically those ethical questions pertinent to the nurse as researcher. Three perspectives of ethical inquiry are identified: that of the nurse, that of the patient and family, and that of the clinical and research environment.

Greene, Maxine. "Ethical Choosing." In Elaine Lynne LaMonica, *The Humanistic Nursing Process*. Monterey, CA: Wadsworth Health Sciences Division, 1985; pp. 270–287.

Griffin, Anne P. "A Philosophical Analysis of Caring in Nursing." *Journal of Advanced Nursing 8* (1983): 289–295.

Guinee, Kathleen K. *The Professional Nurse: Orientation, Roles, and Responsibilities*. London: Macmillan, 1970. 177 pp.

Jameton, Andrew, & Jackson, E. M. "Nuclear War and Nursing Ethics: What Is the Nurse's Responsibility?" *Mobius 4* (1984): 75–88.

Kemp, V. H. "The Role of Critical Care Nurses in the Ethical Decision-Making Process." *Dimensions in Critical Care Nursing 4* (1985): 354–359.

Ketefian, Shake. "A Case Study of Theory Development: Moral Behavior in Nursing." *Advances in Nursing Science 9* (1987): 10–19.

Ketefian, Shake (Ed.). *Ethics for Nursing*. Gaithersburg, MD: Aspen Systems Corp., 1982. 92 pp. (*Topics in Clinical Nursing*; Vol. 4, No. 1)

Lumpp, Francesca. "The Role of the Nurse in the Bioethical Decision-Making Process." In *Nursing Clinics of North America*, Vol. 14, No. 1, March 1979. Philadelphia: W. B. Saunders, 1979; pp. 13–21.

McCloskey, Joanne Comi, & Grace, Helen Kennedy (Eds.). *Current Issues in Nursing* (2nd ed.). Boston: Blackwell Scientific Publications; St. Louis: Distributors, USA, Blackwell Mosby Book Distributors, 1985. 1138 pp.

Midwest Alliance in Nursing. Fall Workshop (6th, 1985, Indianapolis, IN) *Health Care Ethics: Dilemmas, Issues, and Conflicts*, edited by Valencia N. Prock, Barbara B. Minckley, Lu Ann Young; Midwest Alliance in Nursing, Fall Workshop, September 1985. Indianapolis, IN: Midwest Alliance in Nursing, 1986. 144 pp.

Minami, Hiroko. "East Meets West: Some Ethical Considerations." *International Journal of Nursing Studies 22* (1985): 311–318.

Mitchell, Christine. "Integrity in Interprofessional Relationships." In George J. Agich (Ed.), *Responsibility in Health Care*. Boston: D. Reidel, 1982; pp. 163–184.

Muyskens, James L. *Moral Problems in Nursing: A Philosophical Investigation.* Totowa, NJ: Rowman and Littlefield, 1982. 208 pp. (Philosophy and Society.)

National League for Nursing. *Ethical Issues in Nursing and Nursing Education.* New York: National League for Nursing, 1980. 72 pp.

Newton, Lisa H. "To Whom Is the Nurse Accountable? A Philosophical Perspective." *Connecticut Medicine* 43 (1979): 7–9.

Parsons, Sara E. *Nursing Problems and Obligations.* New York: Garland Pub., 1985. 149 pp. (The History of American Nursing series) Reprint originally published by Whitcomb & Barrows (Boston), 1916.

Payton, Rita J. "Pluralistic Ethical Decision Making." In American Nurses' Association, *Divisions on Practice, Clinical and Scientific Sessions, 1979.* St. Louis, MO: American Nurses' Association, 1979; pp. 9–16.

Pinch, W. J. "Ethical Dilemmas in Nursing: The Role of the Nurse and Perceptions of Autonomy." *Journal of Nursing Education* 24 (1985): 372–376.

Poletti, R. A. "Ethics of Death and Dying." *International Journal of Nursing Studies* 22 (1985): 329–334.

Pyne, Reginald H. *Professional Discipline in Nursing: Theory and Practice.* Oxford; Boston: Blackwell Scientific Publications; St. Louis, MO: Blackwell Mosby Book Distributors, 1981. 160 pp.

Quinn, Carroll A., & Smith, Michael D. *The Professional Commitment: Issues and Ethics in Nursing.* Philadelphia: Saunders, 1987. 188 pp. Although this work does not claim that nursing is a profession, it addresses the ethical implications of such a claim. Following an introduction to basic principles of ethics, specific issues—such as the professional–professional relationship and collective action—are discussed.

Shannon, Thomas A. "Nursing Ethics: Duties and Dilemmas." In *Twelve Problems in Health Care Ethics.* Lewiston, NY: E. Mellen Press; 1984: pp. 271–307.

Sigman, Paula. "Ethical Choice in Nursing." *Advances in Nursing Science 1* (1979): 37–52.

Spicker, Stuart F., & Gadow, Sally (Eds.). *Nursing: Images and Ideals; Opening Dialogue with the Humanities.* New York: Springer, 1980. 193 pp. Selected essays based upon a November 1977 conference convened by the Committee on Philosophy and Medicine, American Philosophical Association address the "fractured image" of the contemporary nurse as well as the philosophical ideals of the nursing profession.

Steele, Shirley M., & Harmon, Vera M. *Values Clarification in Nursing* (2nd ed.). Norwalk, CT: Appleton–Century–Crofts, 1983. 225 pp.

Stenberg, Marjorie J. "The Search for a Conceptual Framework as a Philosophic Basis for Nursing Ethics: An Examination of Code, Contract, Context, and Covenant." *Military Medicine* 144 (1979): 9–22.

Storch, J. *Patient's Rights: Ethical and Legal Issues in Health Care and Nursing.* Toronto: McGraw–Hill Ryerson, 1982. 288 pp.

Theis, E. C. "Ethical Issues: A Nursing Perspective." *New England Journal of Medicine* 315 (1986): 1222–1224.

Thompson, Ian E.; Melia, Kath M.; and Boyd, Kenneth M. *Nursing Ethics.*

Edinburgh; New York: Churchill Livingstone, 1983. 143 pp. The joint effort of a nurse, a philosopher, and a theologian, this work presents varied perspectives on moral dilemmas in nursing.

Thompson, Joyce Beebe, & Thompson, Henry O. *Bioethical Decision Making for Nurses.* Norwalk, CT: Appleton–Century–Crofts, 1985. 253 pp. Following an overview of the theoretical bases for bioethics, the authors present their ten-step model for bioethical decision making.

Thompson, Joyce Beebe, & Thompson, Henry O. *Ethics in Nursing.* New York: Macmillan, 1981. 258 pp. Intended as a textbook for nursing students, this work presents clusters of bioethical issues pertinent to various stages in the human life cycle beginning with genetics and ending with the elderly. Brief case studies as well as extended footnotes are provided.

Trandel-Korenchuk, D. M., & Trandel-Korenchuk, K. M. "Disclosure of Information in Nursing." *Nursing Administration Quarterly* 10 (1986): 69–73.

Veatch, Robert M., & Fry, Sara T. *Case Studies in Nursing Ethics.* Philadelphia: Lippincott, 1987. 312 pp.

Wilson-Barnett, Jenifer. "Ethical Dilemmas in Nursing." *Journal of Medical Ethics* 12 (1986): 123–126, 135.

Winslow, Gerald R. "From Loyalty to Advocacy: A New Metaphor for Nursing." *Hastings Center Report* 14 (1984): 32–40.

Woodruff, A. M. "Becoming a Nurse: The Ethical Perspective." *International Journal of Nursing Studies* 22 (1985): 295–302.

Wright, Richard A. *Human Values in Health Care: The Practice of Ethics.* New York: McGraw–Hill, 1987. 303 pp. A multi-faceted work, this book provides a theoretical introduction to ethical decision making for health care professionals, 14 selected essays, and an appendix of selected professional codes of ethics.

Yarling, R. R., & McElmurry, B. J. "The Moral Foundations of Nursing." *Advances in Nursing Science* 8 (1986): 63–73.

Codes of the Nursing Profession

American Association of Occupational Health Nurses. "American Association of Occupational Health Nurses Code of Ethics." *Occupational Health Nursing* 25 (1977): 28.

American Nurses' Association. *Code for Nurses with Interpretive Statements.* Kansas City, MO: The Association, 1985. 16 pp.

American Nurses' Association. *Human Rights Guidelines for Nurses in Clinical and Other Research.* Kansas City, MO. (2420 Pershing Rd., Kansas City, MO 64108): The Association, 1985. Revised edition of *Human Rights Guidelines for Nurses in Clinical and Other Research* prepared by Jeanne Quint Benoliel and Jeanne S. Berthold, 1975. 16 pp.

American Nurses' Association. *The Nurse in Research: ANA Guidelines on Ethical Values.* New York, 1968. 6 pp.

American Nurses' Association. *Nursing: A Social Policy Statement.* Kansas City, MO: The Association, 1980.

American Nurses' Association. *Perspectives on the Code for Nurses.* Kansas City, MO: The Association, 1978. 60 pp. The perspectives provided are those of the historian, the educator, the practicing nurse, the nurse administrator, the researcher, and the philosopher. The papers included were originally presented at the ANA Convention in Atlantic City, NJ, June 1976.

American Nurses' Association. *Committee on Ethical, Legal and Professional Standards. Code for Nurses with Interpretive Statements.* New York [1968] 1 vol. (unpaged)

American Nurses' Association. *Committee on Ethics. Guidelines for Implementing the Code for Nurses.* Kansas City, MO: The Association, 1980. Code for nurses was developed by the American Nurses' Association Committee on Ethical, Legal and Professional Standards.

Canadian Nurses Association. *CNA Code of Ethics: An Ethical Basis for Nursing in Canada.* Ottawa: Canadian Nurses Association, February 1980. 6 pp.

Canadian Nurses Association. *CNA Code of Ethics.* Ottawa: Canadian Nurses Association, 1985.

Canadian Nurses Association. *Ethical Guidelines for Nursing Research Involving Human Subjects.* Ottawa: Canadian Nurses Association, 1983.

Canadian Nurses Association, Canadian Medical Association, & Canadian Hospital Association. "Joint Statement on Terminal Illness: A Protocol for Health Professionals Regarding Resuscitative Intervention for the Terminally Ill." Ottawa: Canadian Nurses Association, 1983.

Flaherty, M. Josephine. "Two Canadian Nursing Codes." *Westminster Institute Review 1* (1981): 11.

Hull, Richard T. "The Function of Professional Codes of Ethics." *Westminster Institute Review 1* (1981): 12–13.

"ICN Nurses' Code." *Australian Nurses' Journal 3* (1973): 17+.

International Council of Nurses. *Code for Nurses: Ethical Concepts Applied to Nursing.* Geneva, Switzerland: The Council, 1973.

Mannino, M. J. "The AANA Code of Ethics." *AANA Journal 54* (1986): 473–475.

Martinson, Ida M. "Confidentiality Pledge for Research Grant Staff." *Nursing Research 29* (1980): 261–262.

Mitchell, D., and Morton, A. "Code of Controversy? UKCC Code of Professional Conduct." *Nursing Mirror 157* (1983): 11–13 pp.

Royal College of Nursing of the United Kingdom. *Guidelines on Confidentiality in Nursing.* London: The College, 1980. 14 pp. Cognizant of the fact that nurses deal with a greatly expanded group of people having access to confidential information, the Royal College developed these guidelines to help the nurse protect the confidentiality of patient information.

Royal College of Nursing (RCN) Code of Professional Conduct: A Discussion Document." *Journal of Medical Ethics 3* (1977): 115–123.

"Second Edition of UKCC Code Published." *Nursing Standard 363* (1984): 1.

Silva, Mary Cipriano. "The American Nurses' Association's Code for Nurses: Purposes, Content, and Enforceability." *Health Matrix 2* (1984): 55–63.

Silva, Mary Cipriano. "The American Nurses' Association's Position Statement

on Nursing and Social Policy: Philosophical and Ethical Dimensions."
Journal of Advanced Nursing 8 (1983): 147–151.

Sward, Kathleen M. "The Code for Nurses: A Guide for Ethical Nursing Practice." *Journal of the New York State Nurses Association 6* (1975): 25–32.

Thompson, H. O., & Thompson, J. E. "Code of Ethics for Nurse-Midwives." *Journal of Nurse-Midwifery 31* (1986): 99–102.

Wilson, Jane. "A New Code of Ethics for Nursing." *Canadian Medical Association Journal 130* (1984); 920–921.

Yeaworth, Rosalee C. "The ANA Code: A Comparative Perspective." *Image: The Journal of Nursing Scholarship 17* (1985): 94–98.

Ethics and Nursing Education

Applegate, Minerva, L., & Entrekin, Nina M. *Teaching Ethics in Nursing: A Handbook for Use of the Case-Study Approach.* New York: National League for Nursing, 1984. 81 pp. Designed for use with *Case Studies for Students: A Companion to Teaching Ethics in Nursing,* this booklet includes introductory material to aid the instructor. Twelve case studies are provided for discussion. (*Case Studies . . . ,* only 36 pages in length, is intended as the resource for the student.)

Berkowitz, Marvin W. "The Role of Discussion in Ethics Training." *Topics in Clinical Nursing 4* (1982): 33–48.

Bridston, Elizabeth O. "An Educational Strategy for Enhancement of Moral-Ethical Decision Making." *Topics in Clinical Nursing 4* (1982): 57–65.

Fromer, Margot Joan. "Teaching Ethics by Case Analysis." *Nursing Outlook 28* (1980): 604–609.

Gilbert, Carol. "The What and How of Ethics Education." *Topics in Clinical Nursing 4* (1982): 49–56.

Kellmer, Dorothy M. "The Teaching of Ethical Decision-Making in Schools of Nursing." *Nursing Leadership 5* (1982): 20–26.

Killeen, M. L. "Nursing Fundamentals Texts: Where's the Ethics?" *Journal of Nursing Education 25* (1986): 334–340.

Reich, Warren T. "A Laboratory for Humanities and the Health Professions." *Mobius 2* (1983): 61–71.

Smith, S. J., & Davis, A. J. "A Programme for Nursing Ethics." *International Journal of Nursing Studies 22* (1985): 335–339.

Stanley, A. Theresa. "Ethics in Nursing Practice and Education: Curriculum Considerations." *American Nurses' Association Publication G–145* (1980): 39–52.

Stenberg, Marjorie J. "Ethics as a Component of Nursing Education." *Advances in Nursing Science 1* (1979): 53–61.

Swider, S. M.; McElmurry, B. J.; & Yarling, R. R. "Ethical Decision Making in a Bureaucratic Context by Senior Nursing Students." *Nursing Research 34* (1985): 108–112.

Ethics and Nursing Practice

Aroskar, Mila A. "Are Nurses' Mind Sets Compatible with Ethical Practice?" *Topics in Clinical Nursing 4* (1982): 22–32.

Aroskar, Mila A. "Ethical Issues in Community Health Nursing." In *Nursing Clinics of North America*, Vol. 14, No. 1, March 1979. Philadelphia: W. B. Saunders, 1979; pp. 35–44.

Benjamin, Martin, & Curtis, Joy. "Virtue and the Practice of Nursing." In Earl E. Shelp (Ed.), *Virtue and Medicine: Explorations in the Character of Medicine.* Boston: D. Reidel, 1985; pp. 257–274.

Bishop, Anne H., & Scudder, John R., Jr. (Eds.). *Caring, Curing, Coping: Nurse, Physician, Patient Relationships.* University, AL: University of Alabama Press, 1985. 130 pp. Papers presented at the Conference "Coping, Curing, Caring: Patient, Physician, Nurse Relationships, held April 8–9, 1983, in Lynchburg, VA, and sponsored by the Departments of Philosophy and Nursing at Lynchburg College.

Campbell, Alastair V. *Moral Dilemmas in Medicine: A Coursebook in Ethics for Doctors and Nurses.* Baltimore: Williams & Wilkins, 1972. 214 pp.

Clatterbuck, Sandra Eller, & Proulx, Joseph R. *A Framework for Ethical Action in Nursing Service Administration.* New York: National League for Nursing, 1981. 28 pp. (League Exchange; No. 128). One of few writings geared toward the nurse administrator, this pamphlet provides a brief introduction to the development of an ethical power base.

Curtin, Leah. "Autonomy, Accountability and Nursing Practice." *Topics in Clinical Nursing 4* (1982): 7–14.

Davis, Anne J. "Ethics and Nursing Administration." In N. L. Chaska (Ed.). *The Nursing Profession: A Time to Speak.* New York: McGraw–Hill, 1982, pp. 650–658.

Davis, Anne J., & Aroskar, Mila A. *Ethical Dilemmas and Nursing Practice* (2nd ed.). Norwalk, CT: Appleton–Century–Crofts, 1983. 243 pp. The first five chapters provide a basic understanding of health care ethics, moral development, selected approaches and principles in ethics, and the constraints upon the nurse in an institutional setting. Then ethical issues in six areas of health care (such as behavior control and informed consent) are examined. Pertinent case studies suitable for class discussion are provided.

DeJoseph, Jeanne F. "Creating a Nursing Ethics Committee: Content and Process." *Perioperative Nursing Quarterly 2* (1986): 42–47.

Donovan, Constance T. "Toward a Nursing Ethics Program in an Acute Care Setting." *Topics in Clinical Nursing 5* (1983): 55–62.

Drane, James F. "Ethics and Nurse Anesthetists: Part I." *Journal of the American Association of Nurse Anesthetists 51* (1983): 48–54.

Drane, James F. "Ethics and Nurse Anesthetists: Part II." *Journal of the American Association of Nurse Anesthetists 51* (1983): 159–166.

Ellison, P., & Walwork, E. "Withdrawing Mechanical Support from the Brain-Damaged Neonate." *Dimensions in Critical Care Nursing 5* (1986): 284–293.

Fowler, Marsha D. M., & Levine-Ariff, June (Eds.). *Ethics at the Bedside: A Source Book for the Critical Care Nurse.* Philadelphia: Lippincott, 1987. 270 pp.

Fromer, Margot Joan. "Solving Ethical Dilemmas in Nursing Practice." *Topics in Clinical Nursing* 4 (1982): 15–21.

Fry, Sara T. "Confidentiality in Health Care: A Decrepit Concept?" *Nursing Economic$* 2 (1984): 413–418.

Fry, Sara T. "Ethical Aspects of Decision-Making in the Feeding of Cancer Patients." *Seminars in Oncological Nursing* 2 (1986): 59–62.

Fry, Sara T. "Ethical Inquiry in Nursing: The Definition and Method of Biomedical Ethics (Continuing Education Credit)." *Perioperative Nursing Quarterly* 2 (1986): 1–8.

Fry, Sara T. "Ethics in Community Health Nursing Practice." In Marcia Stanhope and Lancaster, Jeanette (Eds.), *Community Health Nursing: Process and Practice for Promoting Health.* St. Louis, MO: C. V. Mosby, 1984; pp. 77–96.

Fry, Sara T. "Individual vs. Aggregate Good: Ethical Tension in Nursing Practice." *International Journal of Nursing Studies* 22 (1985): 303–310.

Gunter, Laurie M. "Ethical Considerations for Nursing Care of Older Patients in the Acute Care Setting." *Nursing Clinics of North America* 18 (1983): 411–421.

Hirschfeld, J. J. "Ethics and Care for the Elderly." *International Journal of Nursing Studies* 22 (1985): 319–328.

Huckabay, L. M. "Ethical–Moral Issues in Nursing Practice and Decision Making." *Nursing Administration Quarterly* 10 (1986): 61–67.

Jameton, Andrew. *Nursing Practice: The Ethical Issues.* Englewood Cliffs, NJ: Prentice-Hall, 1984. 331 pp. (Prentice-Hall Series in the Philosophy of Medicine)

Kluge, Eike-Henner W. "The Profession of Nursing and the Right to Strike." *Westminster Institute Review* 2 (1982): 3–6.

Lawrence, Jeanette A., & Farr, E. Helen. "The Nurse Should Consider Critical Care Ethical Issues." *Journal of Advanced Nursing* 7 (1982): 223–229.

Murphy, Catherine P., & Hunter, Howard (Eds.). *Ethical Problems in the Nurse–Patient Relationship.* Boston: Allyn and Bacon, 1983. 276 pp. Foundations of the nursing profession, the role of the nurse, and issues in the nurse–patient relationship are addressed in this anthology of original essays. Appendices contain the major codes of ethics relevant to nursing.

Muyskens, James L. "Nurses' Collective Responsibility and the Strike Weapon." *Journal of Medicine and Philosophy* 7 (1982): 101–112.

Nelson, M. Janice. "Authenticity: Fabric of Ethical Nursing Practice." *Topics in Clinical Nursing* 4 (1982): 1–6. *The Nurse's Dilemma: Ethical Considerations in Nursing Practice.* Geneva: International Council of Nurses; New York: printed in U.S. by the American Journal of Nursing Co., 1977. Sponsored by the International Council of Nurses and the Florence Nightingale International Foundation. Project Director: Barbara L. Tate.

Olson, J. "To Treat or to Allow to Die: An Ethical Dilemma in Gerontological Nursing." *Journal of Gerontological Nursing* 7 (1981): 141–144, 147.

Robinson, M. B. "Patient Advocacy and the Nurse: Is There a Conflict of Interest?" *Nursing Forum* 22 (1985): 58–63.

Rumbold, Graham. *Ethics in Nursing Practice.* Philadelphia: Bailliere Tindall, 1986. 160 pp.

Siantz, Mary Lou de Leon (Ed.). *Bioethical Issues in Nursing.* Philadelphia: Saunders, 1979. (*Nursing Clinics of North America*, Vol. 14, No. 1, pp. 1–91.) Contributions by recipients of Kennedy Foundation Fellowships in Medical Ethics for Nursing Faculty focus on ethical problems in nursing specialties (community health, intensive care, terminal care, gerontology) as well as questions relating to moral development and clinical decision making, the nurse's role in decision making, and human values and the care of the mentally retarded.

Sideleau, Barbara Flynn (Ed.). *Ethical Issues in Mental Health Nursing.* New York: McGraw–Hill, 1978. 104 pp.

Silva, Mary Cipriano. "Comprehension of Information for Informed Consent by Spouses of Surgical Patients." *Research in Nursing and Health 8* (1985): 117–124.

Silva, Mary Cipriano. "Ethics, Informed Consent and the OR Nurse." *Todays OR Nurse 4* (1982): 21–22, 24, 62–63.

Silva, Mary Cipriano. "Ethics, Scarce Resources, and the Nurse Executive." *Nursing Economic$ 2* (1984): 11–18.

Storch, Janet L. *Patient's Rights: Ethical and Legal Issues in Health Care and Nursing.* New York: McGraw–Hill Ryerson, 1982. 249 pp. After discussing the substance and origins of patients' rights and their relationship to the law, the author addresses, from a Canadian perspective, the right to be informed, the right to be respected, the right to participate, and the right to equal access to health care.

Yarling, R. R., & McElmurry, B. J. "Rethinking the Nurse's Role in 'Do Not Resuscitate' Orders: A Clinical Policy Proposal in Nursing Ethics." *Advances in Nursing Science 5* (1983): 1–12.

Youell, L. *Major Ethical Problems Faced by Nursing Administrators.* Edmonton: Department of Health Services Administration and Community Medicine, University of Alberta, 1984.

Ethics and Nursing Research

AACN Task Force on Ethics in Critical Care Research. "Part One: Statement on Ethics in Critical Care Research." *Focus on Critical Care 12* (1985): 47–57.

Davis, Anne J. "Ethical Issues in Nursing Research." [Column appearing in *Western Journal of Nursing Research* beginning with Volume 7 (1985)].

Davis, Anne J., & Mahon, Kathleen A. "Research with the Mentally Retarded and Mentally Ill: Rights and Duties Versus Compelling State Interest." *Journal of Advanced Nursing 9* (1984): 15–21.

Fry, Sara T. "Ethics and Nursing Research." *Virginia Nurse 50* (1982): 16–21.

McClowry, S. G. "Research and Treatment: Ethical Distinctions Related to the Care of Children." *Journal of Pediatric Nursing 2* (1987): 23–29.

Munhall, Patricia L. "Ethical Juxtapositions in Nursing Research." *Topics in Clinical Nursing 4* (1982): 66–73.

Royal College of Nursing of the United Kingdom. *Ethics Related to Research in Nursing.* London: Royal College of Nursing of the United Kingdom, 1977.

Scott, Diane W. "Ethical Issues in Nursing Research: Access to Human Subjects." *Topics in Clinical Nursing* 4 (1982): 74–83.

Silva, Mary Cipriano, & Sorrell, J. M. "Factors Influencing Comprehension of Information for Informed Consent: Ethical Implications for Nursing Research." *International Journal of Nursing Studies* 21 (1984): 233–240.

KEEPING UP WITH NEW DEVELOPMENTS IN NURSING ETHICS

As of this writing there are two newsletters devoted to nursing ethics: *Ethics Happenings*, published by the Center for Nursing Ethics, George Mason University, (4400 University Drive, Fairfax, VA 22030) and *Ethical Issues in Nursing*, a bimonthly newsletter produced by the program in Medical Ethics, UCLA Medical Center (Contact: Leslie Steven Rothenberg, Department of Medicine, Division of Pulmonary and Critical Care Medicine, 37–131 CHS, UCLA School of Medicine, Los Angeles, CA 90024). *Ethics Happenings* is oriented toward brief essays, news items regarding the Center for Nursing Ethics and current bibliographic information, whereas *Ethical Issues in Nursing* consists of citations to recent periodical literature on nursing ethics, all of which are accompanied by lengthy, informative annotations.

Comprehensive bibliographical information on nursing ethics and bioethical issues in general is available online by searching the BIOETHICSLINE database (supported and distributed by the National Library of Medicine, Bethesda, MD) and in print by consulting the annual volumes of the *Bibliography of Bioethics* (a publication of the Kennedy Institute of Ethics Information Retrieval Project). For those with access to personal computers, the major search terms to be used are "*nurses" or "*nursing ethics" (each qualified by the use of "(kw)" to indicate that these are terms from the Bioethics Thesaurus, the controlled vocabulary employed to index the BIOETHICSLINE database). There are many ways to expand or restrict a search of the database; consultation on search strategy as well as searches of the database are available from the National Reference Center for Bioethics Literature, Kennedy Institute of Ethics, Georgetown University, Washington, DC 20057, 1–800–MED–ETHX or 202–687–3885.

The preparation of this bibliography was supported in part by funds provided under Grant Number LM04492 from the National Library of Medicine, National Institutes of Health.

Case Examples of Ethical Dilemmas Involving Nurse Administrators

As with the others in this book, the cases presented in Appendix B represent actual ethical dilemmas encountered by nurse administrators who attended the Division of Nursing funded conferences on "Ethical Decision Making for Nurse Executives" from 1984 through June 1989. To facilitate the reader's analyses of the ethical dilemmas, the six cases containing the dilemmas are presented first; outcomes for each case then follow in a separate section so as not to bias the reader. The outcomes described represent actual rather than idealized resolutions.

CASE 1

The Chemically Dependent Nurse[1]

As Director of Nursing, Miss A was informed by a Unit Supervisor that a staff nurse was told by a patient that the nurse who worked the night before awakened her at 3:30 AM and gave her a "double dose" of Demerol that she had not requested. The patient stated that the nurse also gave her roommate an injection at the same time and that the nurse appeared very sleepy. Since the roommate was discharged that morning, she was unable to comment. The staff nurse checked the narcotic sign-out sheet and three doses of demerol had been signed out. The patient did not want the nurse assigned to her.

Miss A and the Unit Supervisor arranged a meeting to review the situation. The nurse in question, Miss B, was oriented two months earlier and was always "buddied" with another nurse until last week. Miss B held a BS in chemistry, an AD in nursing, and had had approximately three months' staff nurse experi-

---

[1]**Case Submitted by:** Helen Wilmarth, RN, MSN, Director Nursing Services, Holy Cross Hospital, Silver Spring, MD.

ence before moving out of state and beginning employment here. It was noted during orientation that she was rather slow and kept to herself.

The Supervisor checked the narcotic sign-out sheets that confirmed the staff nurse's story. She also checked all the sign-out sheets for the past week and found that many doses of demerol were signed out by Miss B. The Supervisor reviewed the patient records and, with the exception of the patient who spoke to the evening nurse, all the others were elderly, were suffering transient confusions, and were given only minimal or no pain medication by other staff nurses. The Supervisor noted that Miss B was not accurate in charting either the patients' responses to the demerol or the times and dates the drug was administered. In addition, Miss B did not follow hospital procedure for "wasting a narcotic."

Questions raised by Miss A and the Supervisor were as follows: If Miss B admits to the evidence, should she remain under close supervision? Should she be terminated? What are the Director's and Supervisor's responsibilities to the hospital? To the nursing profession? To the nurse?

The next day Miss A gave Miss B notice of a formal meeting in which her inability to follow policies and procedures related to administration of narcotics would be discussed. It is hospital practice to give the employee 48 hours notice. Miss B was suspended from work until the scheduled meeting. She left frightened and tearful.

Two days later the facts were reviewed. Miss B became angry and felt she was being accused of something. She did not understand what was written about her performance, so Miss A reviewed individual patient records with her, pointing out the discrepancies. Miss B acknowledged that she was not following procedure. She could not recall what she had done with the "wasted narcotics." She heard the concern the Director had with her assessment skills and her inability to carry out procedures accurately. During the meeting the nurse's speech was slowed and very deliberate. She asked to be given the opportunity to correct her mistakes and return to work immediately. She stated that her father had been through a terminal illness and that she, too, knew what it was like to suffer pain. She wanted to be able to help others. She was told that the final action would be decided within the next two days, and until that time she could not work. (See p. 262 for case outcome.)

A Nurse's Conscientious Refusal to Care for a Patient[1]

Ms D is the Nursing Administrator in a 500-bed university hospital. In one of their regular meetings, the Clinical Director of the Obstetrics and Gynecology Service told Ms D that the Head Nurse on the obstetrics unit had a problem. Ms R, a nurse who has been working in the unit for four months, asked not to be assigned to a patient who was admitted for a second trimester abortion. The Head Nurse arranged the patient's assignment accordingly and then reminded Ms R that she had been informed about the abortions before she accepted employment on the unit. Ms R agreed that she had known but added that she had rethought her position since that time, and she was not comfortable with preparing the medication or being involved in the labor and delivery process. Ms R stated that she had no problem giving care to the patient after delivery and felt she could be supportive during that period. The Head Nurse told Ms R that she would have to consider whether Ms R could maintain her employment or whether she would have to transfer to another unit. Ms R said that she really liked the unit and did not want to transfer; however, she had not changed her mind about assisting with abortions. The Head Nurse discussed it with the Clinical Director, who then asked Ms D's support in transferring Ms R or in asking for her resignation. Ms D asked if there was any way that the unit could accommodate Ms R's convictions. The Clinical Director felt this was not possible, adding that others were not comfortable with the abortions but did work with patients. She wondered if others would ask for special treatment.

Ms D felt a moral conflict in the situation, that is, the right of an individual nurse to refuse in conscience to perform an act versus the responsibility of the Department of Nursing to provide care for the patients within the hospital. She found herself in conflict with her own staff in that she felt accommodation could be made. Could she impose this view on her staff? What if she did and the staff refused to care for these patients? Would she then have violated her obligation to the patients and the institution? (*See* p. 263 for case outcome.)

---

[1]**Case Submitted by: Sheila M. McCarthy, RN, MSN, CNAA,** Director of Nursing, The George Washington University Medical Center, Washington, D.C.

CASE 3

A Nurse Practitioner Disagrees with a Physician's Assessment of a Patient[1]

Dr Y was a contract pediatrician working in the well baby clinic in a local health department. The clinic also was staffed by a pediatric nurse practitioner and public health nurses who are full-time employees of the health department. Since Dr Y began working at the health department, both the nurse practitioner and the public health nurses have expressed concerns about incorrect diagnoses and improper treatment of certain common conditions such as iron deficiency anemia. Additionally, there were concerns that Dr Y was superficial in her examinations.

Baby N was several weeks old and was being followed with weekly weight checks because of his failure to gain weight. Dr Y saw Baby N several weeks in a row but kept bringing him back for yet another weight check instead of referring him for further evaluation. The nurse practitioner felt that the child was ill and needed a thorough workup. Dr Y, however, who ultimately was in charge of the case, felt that the case could be managed in the clinic.

Do the nurses defer to the physician's authority and medical expertise? Or do they find some way to have the child evaluated outside the health department? (*See* p. 263 for case outcome.)

---

[1]Although the nurse administrator and her nursing superior were willing to identify the administrator's name and agency, the Health Director, a physician, refused permission for such identification.

CASE 4

The Marginally Competent Staff Nurse[1]

Mrs M, a staff nurse for 15 years at a county health department, was doing marginal level work. With the guidance of Miss J, the Director of Nursing, the nursing supervisor developed a specific action plan that Mrs M must implement if she wished to continue her employment. Mrs M appealed the plan to

---

[1]Case Submitted by: JoAnne M. Jorgenson, RN, MPH, Director of Nursing Services, Fairfax County Health Department, Fairfax, VA.

Miss J; consequently, a conference was held with all three in attendance. Mrs M denied all problem areas, refuted notes describing conferences held with her, and offered numerous reasons why she couldn't be expected to perform at the level spelled out by her supervisor. A mutually agreed upon plan was developed on an incremental basis with specific time frames for completion. The final outcome remained that Mrs M apply herself or her job would be in jeopardy.

Mrs M was a favorite among her peers in the office. She was the social director, joke teller, first to hear the news, and first to share it. It was not long after the conference that its content was known by her peers—from her perspective.

Miss J received a request from two senior staff in another office to meet with them regarding a personnel matter. During this conference Miss J was advised that staff were very upset and angry about the way Mrs M was being treated. They have learned from Mrs M that she was being forced out with lies, "trumped up charges," and that the administration was trying to get rid of all the "old" nurses who didn't have degrees. Miss J explained that she could not comment on the specifics of Mrs M's evaluation but reassured the two senior staff that there was no plan to in any way remove senior nurses who did not have degrees. Miss J reiterated that these senior nurses are the core of the staff due to their experience and knowledge of the community and health services.

A follow-up conference with Mrs M was held as planned to discuss her work performance evaluation. There was minimal improvement; Mrs M had decided that since the evaluation was not valid, she need not follow through. Miss J firmly spelled out the minimal expectations and gave Mrs M the option to actively fulfill them or make the decision to seek employment elsewhere. A conference was scheduled for two days later, at which time Mrs M was to give her decision. A resignation letter was received by Miss J the next morning.

Mrs M announced her departure to her peers before her supervisor arrived at the office, explaining she was too tired to fight any more. No matter what she did it was not right and the agency was successful in pushing her out. Her peers were upset and hostile when the supervisor arrived.

The supervisor met with Miss J to advise her of the impact of Mrs M's resignation and Mrs M's version of why she was leaving. What do we tell the staff? Do we honor Mrs M's right to a confidential evaluation? Do we try, in some way, to refute the charges being made by staff? Do we let it ride? (*See* p. 264 for case outcome.)

                                              | CASE 5 |

The Operating Room Head Nurse as Witness to Unnecessary Surgery[1]

Mrs F is the Head Nurse of the Operating Room and Recovery Room in a community hospital. She is an excellent nurse who has worked at the hospital for ten years. On a Monday morning Mrs F called for an appointment with the Director of Nursing. When she arrived for her appointment, she was upset about an incident that had occurred over the weekend. It seems that an elderly patient had surgery on the previous Friday, developed complications, and then was subjected to repeated surgeries. Mrs F felt the surgeries were unnecessary and did nothing to improve the patient's quality of life. In addition, Mrs F felt that the patient's family had not been properly informed of the patient's condition and, therefore, were unaware of what was going on. For example, one procedure involved opening a wound in the Intensive Care Unit without any anesthesia or sterility. During this procedure the patient was partially conscious. Mrs F was concerned about how this patient and family, as well as other patients and families under this surgeon's care, could be protected from potential or actual harms. (*See* p. 264 for case outcome.)

---

[1]Case Submitted by: Gail Dempsey Russell, RN, MSN, Vice President/Nursing, Potomac Hospital, Woodbridge, VA.

                                              | CASE 6 |

Nurses' Refusal to Care for AIDS Hospice Patients[1]

The Team Director approached a home care hospice nurse and requested that she admit and follow a patient diagnosed with AIDS. The nurse, however, said that she would be unable to follow this patient because she was trying to get pregnant. Having overheard the conversation, another home care hospice nurse approached the Team Director and also said that she would be unable to care for this patient. She said that her husband was frightened by what he had

---

[1]Case Submitted by: Karen Walborn, RN, MN, Nurse Manager, Hebrew Home of Greater Washington, Rockville, MD.

read about AIDS and had told her that he does not want her caring for AIDS patients. The second nurse said she felt caught between how her husband feels, her own fears about the disease, and her commitment to care for people who are dying. This nurse is a highly respected and committed hospice nurse who regards her current position as "the best job I've ever had"; yet, she states, "I just don't know what to do."

The conflicts perceived are:

1. How can a hospice nurse not care for a dying patient who has AIDS?
2. Does each staff member have the right to refuse to care for a patient with a communicable disease he/she fears?
3. Does the organization have the right to make staff members care for patients with a disease about which more is unknown than is known?

(See p. 264–265 for case outcome.)

Outcomes for Cases in Appendix B

The Chemically Dependent Nurse

The information from the patient, narcotic records, and the results of our discussion were reviewed by the Director of Personnel, the hospital attorney, the hospital Administrator, and the Director. The nurse's negligent practice in administration of narcotics to the patients under her care and her failure to follow established policies and procedures led us to the decision to terminate her employment. As her actions were inconsistent with acceptable practice, we felt legally and morally obligated to report these circumstances to the state licensing board.

Miss A met with the nurse and informed her of the decision to terminate her employment. She also was told that the hospital was obligated to report the circumstances to the state board. Miss A provided Miss B with names of several counseling agencies that would be supportive to her. Miss B expressed feelings of helplessness and failure. She began to hyperventilate and complain of chest pain. Miss A asked her if someone should be called; Miss B asked to go to the Emergency Room. In the Emergency Room she complained of severe chest pain. Her private physician was called and personnel proceeded with her workup. The nurse in charge checked Miss B's former Emergency Room records and discovered she had been there on six previous occasions, and a question of narcotic abuse was noted. On learning that her private physician was arriving, she signed out against medical advice.

Miss A was concerned for her safety but legally could not hold her. The Emergency Room nurses encouraged her to wait, but she denied she needed help and left. She was asked to call Miss A when she got home. She did call. She seemed grateful for the concern for her safety. They discussed her need to see her doctor and to obtain support. She stated she would see her physician and her pastor. About a week later she called once again to say "thank you for all you have done" and to explain she was in counseling.

CASE 2

A Nurse's Conscientious Refusal to Care for a Patient

Ms D discussed the problem with the Clinical Director and the Head Nurse. Together they made a decision. Several resources, including legal counsel, were consulted; however, the decision was made because of ethical, not legal, considerations. The decision was to discuss the problem with the unit staff to see if a nurse could work in the unit and not care for patients having abortions, while as a group the staff had the responsibility to care for all patients including those having abortions. The staff discussion took place. The unit agreed that they had a responsibility as a staff to provide care to all patients on the unit but that they could accommodate among themselves, and Ms R stayed on the unit. Ms R remained on the staff during the next year, and the problem did not arise again.

CASE 3

A Nurse Practitioner Disagrees with a Physician's Assessment of a Patient

When Baby N next came to the clinic, the nurse practitioner saw the infant alone and assessed his condition. She then told Dr Y that she thought the child needed a formal referral for further evaluation and gave her rationale for the decision. Dr Y acquiesced. After clinic, the nurse practitioner met with the physician privately and expressed her concern that the physician had not seen the need for a referral sooner. The doctor countered with a recital of her medical expertise and experience.

Since Dr Y did not admit that she might have made an error in judgment, and in light of other concerns about Dr Y's care, the nurse practitioner and the nursing supervisor together presented the problem to the Health Director, who not only supported the judgment of the nurses, but felt that a Protective Services referral for the family also was in order. He talked with Dr Y about her handling of the case, especially in light of the fact that the child had a severe urinary tract infection. After this incident, concerns about Dr Y continued. Three months later Dr Y was fired by the Health Director.

CASE 4

The Marginally Competent Staff Nurse

Miss J honored the right of Mrs M to a confidential evaluation. After Mrs M's departure, Miss J met with the staff and listened to their concerns, clarifying those areas that could be clarified without violating Mrs M's right to confidentiality. Mrs M requested an appointment with Miss J four months later, at which time she apologized for her behavior, her refusal to look at herself, and thanked the agency for making her realize she needed a change in her employment. She is currently working effectively and happily in a physician's office.

CASE 5

The Operating Room Head Nurse as Witness to Unnecessary Surgery

The Director of Nursing discussed the case with the Chairman of the Surgery Department. After his investigation, the case was presented and thoroughly discussed at a departmental meeting. Following this, a panel of physicians was appointed by the Chief of Staff to review the practice of the surgeon involved.

CASE 6

Nurses' Refusal to Care for AIDS Hospice Patients

The first nurse was not assigned the patient at that time because of her possible pregnancy (she is now pregnant). The second nurse has not been assigned a patient with AIDS yet because there have not been any AIDS patients to care for in her geographical area. Both nurses, however, were reminded that hospice policy in their agency was to care for all patients who meet the admission criteria, regardless of diagnosis, and that the most up-to-date Center for Disease

Control guidelines were being followed. In addition, the Team Director and three other concerned managers requested a meeting with the Assistant Administrator for Patient Services to plan an overall approach to working with patients with AIDS. The outcome of the discussion included the development of an AIDS Task Force composed of representatives from the interdisciplinary team.

Code for Nurses[1]

1 The nurse provides services with respect for human dignity and the uniqueness of the client, unrestricted by considerations of social or economic status, personal attributes, or the nature of health problems.

2 The nurse safeguards the client's right to privacy by judiciously protecting information of a confidential nature.

3 The nurse acts to safeguard the client and the public when health care and safety are affected by the incompetent, unethical, or illegal practice of any person.

4 The nurse assumes responsibility and accountability for individual nursing judgments and actions.

5 The nurse maintains competence in nursing.

6 The nurse exercises informed judgment and uses individual competence and qualifications as criteria in seeking consultation, accepting responsibilities, and delegating nursing activities to others.

7 The nurse participates in activities that contribute to the ongoing development of the profession's body of knowledge.

8 The nurse participates in the profession's efforts to implement and improve standards of nursing.

9 The nurse participates in the profession's efforts to establish and maintain conditions of employment conducive to high quality nursing care.

10 The nurse participates in the profession's effort to protect the public from misinformation and misrepresentation and to maintain the integrity of nursing.

11 The nurse collaborates with members of the health professions and other citizens in promoting community and national efforts to meet the health needs of the public.

[1]**From:** American Nurses' Association. (1985). *Code for nurses with interpretive statements.* Kansas City, MO: Author. Reprinted with permission of the American Nurses' Association.

Index

267